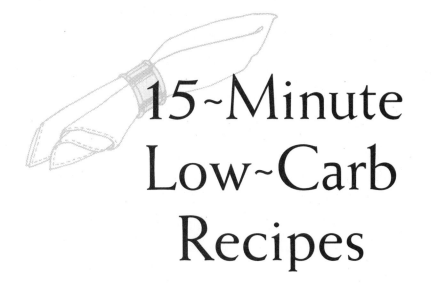

15~Minute Low~Carb Recipes

15~Minute Low~Carb Recipes

INSTANT RECIPES FOR DINNERS, DESSERTS, AND MORE!

Dana Carpender

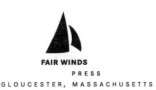

FAIR WINDS
PRESS
GLOUCESTER, MASSACHUSETTS

Text © 2003 by Dana Carpender

First published in the U.S.A. by
Fair Winds Press
33 Commercial Street
Gloucester, Massachusetts 01930-5089

Library of Congress Cataloging-in-Publication Data
Carpender, Dana.
15 minute low-carb recipes : instant recipes for dinners, desserts,
and more! / Dana Carpender.
p. cm.
ISBN 1-59233-041-X
1. Quick and easy cookery. 2. Low-carbohydrate diet—Recipes.
I. Title: Fifteen minute low-carb recipes. II. Title.
TX833.5.C37 2004
641.5'6383--dc22
2003018251

10 9 8 7 6

Cover design by Mary Ann Smith
Design by Leslie Haimes

Printed in Canada

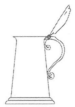

In memory of the late Dr. Robert C. Atkins, 1930–2003.
Because of his fearless tenacity, millions of us live better lives today.

"If I can see far, it is because I have stood on the shoulders of giants."
—Sir Isaac Newton

contents

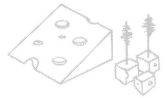

Introduction

Welcome to the world of *15-Minute Low Carb*!

I've known for a long time that, where cooking is concerned, I have a big edge over most of my readers. After all, I work at home. I can put something in the oven an hour or two before dinner, and be here to tend to it if needed. I can simmer a pot of soup all afternoon. I'm here.

Furthermore, at this writing I have no children—only an exceedingly good-tempered and undemanding husband. In short, I never dash in the door at 6:15 p.m., after a long day at the office (and add a few errands on the way home into the bargain), to find people clamoring for me to get dinner on the table as soon as possible, and 5 minutes ago would be nice.

I also never slog home after a 12-hour day, so tired and hungry that the very idea of having to spend an hour getting dinner on the table is enough to send me through the local fast-food drive-in, even without a family to feed.

These are precisely the situations that this book is meant to help you cope with—all while keeping you on your low-carbohydrate diet and making your family happy.

Just What Do I Mean By 15 Minutes?

I mean exactly what I say—that from start to finish, these recipes take 15 minutes or less. I know this for certain because I set the stove timer when I started making them!

Now, it is entirely possible to make these dishes take a little bit longer. For instance, thawing times for frozen foods are not included, so if you haven't thought to take something out of the freezer in the morning, you'll just have to tack on however long it takes your microwave to thaw your food. (This would be a good time to sit down and have a glass of dry wine or a light beer, and maybe put out a tray of veggies and ranch dressing for the troops.) For that matter, more than once I've run two or three minutes over my time limit because I couldn't find the darned Worcestershire sauce or whatever. I take no responsibility for kitchen disorganization, and trust me, I know all about kitchen disorganization. However, once you have your ingredients located, the 15-minute count holds for these recipes, *prep time included*.

This, of course, rules out a fair number of dishes. You'll find no roasts in this book, no meat loaves—indeed, nothing that is cooked in an oven, because even if a dish requires less than 15 minutes in your oven, the preheating time is an obstacle. While there are wonderful soups, there are none of the traditional long-simmered variety. Indeed, you'll find that a few methods of cooking are used over and over, simply because they are speedy—sautéing, stir-frying, grilling, broiling, and microwaving.

You'll find that these recipes generally call for foods, especially meat and poultry, to be thinly cut, sliced, shredded, ground, or cubed. There's no mystery why: The smaller the pieces, the faster the cooking time! Thinly cut pork chops—about 1/4 inch (5 mm) thick—will cook within our time limit. Inch-thick (2 cm) pork chops, however, will not, no matter how juicy and delicious they may be. So if you're in doubt as you cut, chop, or slice your foods up, think "smaller is better."

You'll also find that these recipes call for you to multitask. Quite often I'll tell you to start one component of the dish cooking, then use that cooking time to cut up or measure and mix other ingredients. It's not hard, really—it's just making the best use of your time. Always give the directions a quick read before you go prepping everything in the ingredients list; you might find that there's a perfect time for chopping up veggies and the like without adding a second to your overall preparation and cooking time.

Low~Carb Menu Planning and One~Dish Meals

In the vast majority of the dishes in this book, the biggest source of carbohydrates is vegetables. I trust we can agree that this is the healthiest possible source of carbohydrates, no? Vegetables, however, are more than that—they are the most flavorful source of carbohydrates in our diet, and by cooking our very low-carb proteins with a variety of vegetables, we can create a widely varied, delicious, exciting low-carb cuisine. However, this will sometimes mean that your carbohydrate allowance for a given meal is completely used up by the vegetables in your soup or skillet supper. This, then, becomes a classic one-dish meal, and a beautiful thing it is.

What about My Carb-Eating Family?

No reason not to serve a carbohydrate food on the side, if your family will be bereft without it. However, I must say that many of the quickest, easiest carbohydrate side dishes—instant mashed potatoes, quick-cooking rice, whack-em-on-the-counter biscuits and rolls—are just as processed and nutrient-depleted as they can be, and are also among the carbohydrates with the highest, most devastating blood sugar impact. Better to serve whole-wheat pita bread; corn or whole-wheat tortillas; one of the less damaging pastas (Jerusalem artichoke pasta, widely available at health food stores, has a relatively modest blood sugar impact and tastes like "regular" pasta); or potatoes you've cut into wedges, sprinkled with olive oil, and roasted in your toaster oven for about 15 minutes at 400°F (200°C/Gas Mark 6). If your family loves rice, well, brown rice is *hugely* superior to white rice, let alone Minute Rice, but it's nobody's idea of a 15-minute food. However, it reheats beautifully in the microwave. You could make a good-size pot of it over the weekend, stash it in the refrigerator, and use it later in the week. When you need it, just spoon out however much your family will need for the meal at hand, put it in a covered microwaveable container with a tablespoon or so of water, and nuke it on 70 percent power for a few minutes.

Anyway, the point is that if your family simply *insists* on a concentrated carbohydrate, serve it on the side. And because you love them, make it one of the less processed, less damaging carbohydrates.

What's a "Serving"?

I've gotten a couple of queries from folks who bought *500 Low-Carb Recipes* and want to know how big a serving size is, so I thought I'd better address the matter.

To be quite honest, folks, there's no great technical determination going on here. For the most part, a "serving" is based on what I think would make a reasonable portion, depending on the carbohydrate count, how rich the dish is, and, for main dishes, the protein count. You just divide the dish up into however many portions the recipe says, and you can figure the carb counts on the recipes are accurate. In some cases I've given you a range —"3 or 4 servings," or whatever. In those cases, I've told you how many servings the carb counts are based on, and you can do a little quick mental estimating if, say, you're serving 4 people when I've given the count for 3.

Of course, this "serving" thing is flukey. People are different sizes and have different appetites. For all I know, you have three children under 5 who might reasonably split one adult-size portion. On the other hand, you might have one 17-year-old boy who's shot up from 5'5" to 6'3" in the past year, and what looks like 4 servings to me will be a quick snack for him. You'll just have to eyeball what fraction of the whole dish you're eating, and go from there.

I've had a few people tell me they'd rather have specific serving sizes—like "1 cup" or the like. I see a few problems with this. First of all, it sure won't work with things like steak or chops—I'd have to use weights, instead, and then all my readers would have to run out and buy scales. Secondly, my recipes generally call for things like, "1/2 head cauliflower" or "2 stalks celery." These things vary in size a bit, and as a result yield will fluctuate a bit, too. Also, if one of my recipes calls for "1 1/2 pounds (750 g) boneless, skinless chicken breasts" and your package is labeled "1.65 pounds (700g)," I don't expect you to whack off the difference to get the portions exact.

In short, I hate to have to weigh and measure everything, and I'm betting that a majority of my readers feel the same way, even if some do not. So I apologize to those who like exact measures, but this is how it's going to be for now, at any rate.

What's With the Info about Stuff other than Carbs and Protein?

You'll notice that in places in this book I've included notes regarding other nutritional components of some of the recipes. Most notably, I've included the calorie count if it seems quite low and the calcium or potassium count if it seems quite high. The reason for this is simple: Many people are trying to watch their calories as well as their carbs, and calling their attention to those dishes in this book that are particularly low in calories seemed helpful. Likewise, my e-mail tells me that the two nutrients low-carbers are most concerned they're *not* getting are calcium and potassium. So letting you know when a recipe is a good source of these nutrients also seemed helpful.

All of the recipes do, of course, include the carbohydrate, fiber, usable carbs, and protein counts.

On the Importance of Reading Labels

Do yourself a favor and get in the habit of reading the label on every food product, and I do mean every food product, that has one. I have learned from long, hard, repetitive experience that food processors can, will, and do put sugar, corn syrup, corn starch, and other nutritionally empty, carb-filled garbage into every conceivable food product. You will shave untold thousands of grams of carbohydrates off your intake over the course of a year by simply looking for the product that has *no added junk.*

There are also a good many classes of food products out there to which sugar is virtually always added—the cured meats immediately come to mind. There is almost always sugar in sausage, ham, bacon, hot dogs, liverwurst, and the like. You will look in vain for sugarless varieties of these products. However, you will find that there is quite a range of carb counts because some manufacturers add more sugar than others. I have seen ham that has 1 gram of carbohydrates per serving, and I have seen ham that has 6 grams of carbohydrates per serving—that's a 600 percent difference! Likewise, I've seen hot dogs that have 1 gram of carbohydrates apiece, and I've seen hot dogs that have 5 grams of carbohydrates apiece.

If you're in a position where you can't read the labels—for instance, at the deli counter at the grocery store—then ask questions. The nice deli folks will be glad to read the labels on the ham and salami for you, and they can tell you what goes into the various items they make themselves. You'll want to ask at the meat counter, too, if you're buying something they've mixed up themselves—Italian sausage, marinated meats, or whatever. I have found that if I state simply that I have a medical condition that requires that I be very careful about my diet—and I don't show up at the busiest hour of the week!—folks are generally very nice about this sort of thing.

In short, become a food sleuth. After all, you're paying your hard-earned money for this stuff, and it is quite literally going to become a part of you. Pay at least as much attention to your food shopping as you would if you were buying a car or a computer!

Appliances for 15-Minute Meals

There are a few kitchen appliances that you'll use over and over to make the recipes in this book. They're all quite common, and I feel safe in assuming that the majority of you have most, if not all, of these appliances.

A microwave oven. Surely everybody is clear by now on how quickly these both thaw and cook all sorts of things. We'll use your microwave over and over again to cook one part of a dish while another part is on the stove—to heat a broth, steam a vegetable, or cook the bacon that we're going to use as a topping.

It is assumed in these recipes that you have a microwave oven with a turntable; most of them have been made this way for quite a while now. If your microwave doesn't have a turntable, you'll have to interrupt whatever else you're doing and turn your food a few times during its microwaving time to avoid uneven cooking.

Also, be aware that microwaves vary in power, and my suggestions for power settings and times are therefore approximate. You'll learn pretty quickly whether your microwave is about the same power as mine, or stronger or weaker.

One quick note about thawing things in the microwave: If you're coming home and pulling something right out of the freezer, you'll probably use the microwave to thaw it, and that's fine. However, if you can think of what you'd like to eat ahead of time, you can thaw in the fridge, or even on the counter. (Wrap things in several layers of old newspaper if you're going to be gone for many hours and the day is warm. This will help keep things from going beyond thawing to spoiling.)

A good compromise is to thaw things most of the way in the microwave and then let them finish at room temperature. You retain more juices this way, but sometimes there's just no time for this.

A blender. You'll use this once in a while to puree something. You could probably use a food processor, instead. For that matter, while I use a standard-issue blender with a jar, there's no reason not to use one of those hand-held blenders.

A food processor. Chopping, grinding, and shredding ingredients by hand just doesn't fit into our time frame, in many cases. If you don't yet own a food processor, a simple one that has an S-blade, plus a single disc that slices on one side and shreds on the other, shouldn't set you back more than $50 to $75.

An electric tabletop grill. Made popular by former Heavyweight Champion George Foreman, these appliances are everywhere. Mr. Foreman's version is quite good, but you can buy a cheaper version for all of 20 bucks. The burger chapter of this book assumes you have one of these appliances, but you can cook your burgers in a skillet instead, or in some cases under the broiler. However, since these methods don't cook from both sides at once, you'll spend a few more minutes cooking this way than you would with the grill.

A slow cooker. What, I hear you cry, is a slow cooker doing in a book of *fast* recipes? Answering reader demand, that's what! I've gotten bunches of requests for slow cooker recipes from readers. Obviously, none of the slow cooker recipes will be done in 15 minutes. Instead, they require 15 minutes or less *prep time*, and that's including both the time to assemble the ingredients in the pot and the time to finish the dish and get it on the table when you get home.

If you don't have a slow cooker, consider picking one up. They're not expensive, and I see perfectly good ones all the time at thrift shops and yard sales for next to nothing. Keep your eyes open.

Techniques

There are just a few techniques that will help you get these recipes done in 15 minutes or less.

The Tilted Lid. Many of these recipes are cooked in a skillet. Covering the skillet will speed up cooking, but it also holds in moisture, which is not always what we want. Therefore, I sometimes use the "tilted lid" technique: I put the lid on the skillet but tilt it slightly to one side, leaving about a 1/2-inch (1 cm) gap. This allows steam to escape, while still holding some heat in the pan. When I refer in a recipe to putting a "tilted lid" on the pan, this is what I mean. This is a good technique to use any time you want to speed up a skillet recipe without holding in moisture.

Pounding Meat. It takes only a half a minute or so to beat a boneless, skinless chicken breast or a piece of pork loin until it's 1/2 to 1/4 (10 to 15 mm) inch thick all over, and it cuts a good 5 to 10 minutes off the cooking time—a worthwhile tradeoff. Pounding meat is very easy to do. You just put your chicken breast or piece of pork loin or whatever in a heavy zipper-lock plastic bag, press out the air, and seal it. Then, using any heavy object—a hammer, a dumbbell, an actual meat-pounding device—you pound the sucker all over with barely controlled ferocity (you want to use a tiny bit of control, or you'll pound right through it) until it's a thin sheet of meat. This technique also tenderizes the meat nicely. Once you've done this a time or two, you'll wonder why you haven't been doing it all along.

Guar or Xanthan Shaker. You'll find a description of these ingredients a little further on—they're thickeners, and they're very useful for replacing flour and cornstarch in gravies and sauces.

In *500 Low-Carb Recipes* I recommended always putting guar or xanthan through your blender with part of the liquid to be thickened, so you could avoid lumps. You may now happily forget that technique. Instead, acquire an extra salt shaker, and fill it with guar or xanthan. This will live next to your stove. Whenever you want to thicken a dish, simply sprinkle guar or xanthan over the top of the dish to be thickened, a little at a time, stirring madly all the while (preferably with a whisk). Stop when the dish is just a little less thick than you'd like it to be, as these thickeners will thicken a little more on standing. This works nicely, is worlds easier than transferring stuff into the blender, and doesn't leave you with a blender to wash!

Ice Cube Preservation. This isn't a cooking technique, it's a money-saving technique. A lot of these recipes call for small quantities of things which, in large quantities, would make the dish too high-carb for us—1/2 cup (100 ml) of spaghetti sauce, 1/4 cup (50 ml) of canned crushed pineapple, 2 tablespoons of tomato paste, that sort of thing. I don't know about you, but I'm not about to let the leftovers of those ingredients grow fur in the back of my fridge, only to be thrown away. So I spoon the remainder of the contents into ice cube trays, freeze the resulting spaghetti sauce cubes or pineapple cubes or whatever, pop 'em out, and store 'em in zipper-lock bags in the freezer. That way, the next time I want to use that ingredient, I can thaw just the little bit I need.

Convenience Foods

In this book I have made more liberal use of convenience foods than I normally do. As to the availability of these ingredients, I figured if I could get it in Bloomington, Indiana—a southern Indiana town of 65,000 people—it would be available to a majority of my readers, at least in the United States. You will find that these recipes call for all of the following.

Bagged salad. Where in *500 Low-Carb Recipes* I would have told you to shred half a head of cabbage, in this book I tell you to use bagged coleslaw mix.

Instead of washing fresh spinach (which can often take three or four washings), I've used bagged baby or triple-washed spinach. Mixed greens, European blends—all kinds of bagged salads show up in this book.

Bottled salad dressings. I've used bottled vinaigrette, ranch, Italian, blue cheese, and Caesar dressings in these recipes. These varieties of salad dressings are pretty reliably low-carb, but read the labels to find the brand with the lowest carb count. And this may be just my bias, but I think Paul Newman's salad dressings are excellent.

Chili garlic paste. This is actually a traditional Asian ingredient, consisting mostly, as the name strongly implies, of hot chilies and garlic. This seasoning saves lots of time when we want a recipe to be both hotly spicy and garlicky. Chili garlic paste comes in jars and keeps for months in the refrigerator. It's worth seeking out at Asian markets or particularly comprehensive grocery stores.

Crushed pork rinds. You can purchase pork rind crumbs, if you like—Katiedid's Pork Rinds sells them online (www.geocities.com/lcporkrinds). However, you can make crushed pork rinds very easily: Simply pour a bag of pork rinds into your food processor with the S-blade in place, and run it until you have something the consistency of bread crumbs. Store in a tightly closed container in the refrigerator. I like to have both plain and barbecue-flavor crushed pork rinds on hand.

Frozen vegetables. Because they're already prepped and ready to go, frozen vegetables save a great deal of time in some of these recipes—for instance, trimming and cutting up green beans would take up most of our 15-minute time limit, while you can pour a bag of frozen green beans into a microwaveable container and start them cooking in less than a minute.

I've also used some vegetable blends in this book. This is a great way to get a variety of vegetables in a dish with no extra work.

Jarred Alfredo sauce. This is a nice ingredient for making simple meat and vegetables into a skillet supper, and it's usually lower carb than tomato-based spaghetti sauce. Read your labels, of course, to find the lowest-carbohydrate brand.

Jarred, grated gingerroot. Grated gingerroot is an extraordinary spice. Dried, ground ginger is no substitute, and for this reason I have long kept a gingerroot in a zipper-lock bag in my freezer, ever-ready for grating or mincing. However, this does take at least a few precious minutes. Fortunately grated gingerroot in oil, put up in jars, is now widely available. I have used this prepared grated gingerroot in testing these recipes, and like it so much that I may keep on using it now that this book is done!

If you can't find grated gingerroot in jars, I see no reason not to buy a fresh gingerroot, peel it, and run it through the shredding blade of your food processor, then chop the resulting shreds still further with your S-blade. (Don't grate up more gingerroot than you can use in a few weeks, though; it's best when it's fresh.) Spoon the resulting paste into a jar with a tight lid, add enough canola, peanut, or sunflower oil to cover, and store in the fridge. This will give you grated gingerroot at your fingertips.

Jarred minced garlic. Truth to tell, I greatly prefer fresh garlic, freshly crushed, over any possible substitute. But jarred, minced garlic in oil is very popular and widely available—and it is, no doubt, quicker than crushing fresh garlic, by at least a minute or two. Therefore, I have used jarred, minced garlic in these recipes. I have, however, always given the equivalent measure of fresh garlic, should you, like me, prefer it enough to be willing to take the extra few seconds.

Low~carbohydrate tortillas. La Tortilla Factory makes these, and they're becoming easier and easier to find—I know of at least two stores here in Bloomington that carry them. (For you locals, they're Bloomingfoods and Sahara Mart.) If you can't find these locally, you could ask your local health food store to special-order them for you. There are also a reasonable number of "e-tailers"—online retailers—who offer these.

Low~sugar or no~sugar barbecue sauce and ketchup. There are a number of these on the market; look around or check the e-tailers. However, I have also included recipes for both of these in the Condiments, Sauces, Dressings, and Seasonings chapter of this book (see page 211). They're very useful to have on hand.

Low~sugar preserves. In particular, I find low-sugar apricot preserves to be a wonderfully versatile ingredient. I buy Smucker's brand, and I like it very much. This is lower in sugar by *far* than "all fruit" preserves, which replace sugar with concentrated fruit juice. Folks, sugar from fruit juice is still sugar.

Smucker's also makes artificially sweetened preserves, but they only have about 1 fewer gram of carbohydrates per serving than the low-sugar variety, and many people prefer to avoid aspartame, so I use the low-sugar variety.

Shredded cheese. Virtually every grocery store in America carries shredded cheddar, Monterey Jack, mozzarella, Mexican blend, and the like. When this book calls for shredded cheese, I'm assuming you bought it that way. I'm also assuming that if a recipe calls for crumbled blue cheese, you bought it crumbled.

Sliced mushrooms. A couple of years ago I discovered that my local grocery stores had started selling fresh mushrooms already sliced for the same price as unsliced mushrooms. I never looked back! Whenever a recipe calls for sliced mushrooms, I'm assuming that you bought them already sliced.

Sprinkle-on seasoning blends. There are some recipes for these in the Condiments, Sauces, Dressings, and Seasonings chapter (see page 211), but I've also used some store-bought seasoning blends, all of which are widely available—lemon pepper, Old Bay seasoning, Creole seasoning, barbecue dry-rub seasoning (sometimes called "soul" seasoning), and a wonderful Rosemary-Ginger Rub from Stubb's, of Austin Texas. (Indeed, everything from Stubb's is great, and every product of theirs that I've tried has been lower in sugar than the run-of-the-mill.)

Tapenade. Tapenade is a wonderful relish or spread made mostly of chopped olives. While it's traditionally spread on bread, it adds an exciting flavor to several recipes in this book but saves you the work of chopping up olives, onions, and various other things. Look for tapenade in jars in your grocery store—it will usually be with the olives and pickles, but it might be in the International section, instead.

Basic Ingredients

These are some ingredients I consider standards for low-carb cooking in general—those of you who have read *500 Low-Carb Recipes* may notice these descriptions are familiar.

Avocados. Several recipes in this book call for avocados. Be aware that the little, black, rough-skinned avocados are far lower in carbohydrates (and higher in healthy monounsaturated fat) than the big green ones. All nutritional analyses were done assuming you used little black avocados.

Beer. One or two recipes in this book call for beer. The lowest carbohydrate beers on the market at this writing are Michelob Ultra (2.8 grams per bottle) and Miller Lite and Milwaukee's Best Light (both 3.5 grams per can). These are what I recommend you use. They are also what I recommend you drink, if you're a beer fan.

Blackstrap molasses. What the heck is molasses doing in a low-carb cookbook? It's practically all carbohydrates, after all! Well yes, but I've found that combining Splenda with a very small amount of molasses gives a good, brown-sugar flavor to all sorts of recipes. Always use the darkest molasses you can find—the darker it is, the stronger the flavor and the lower the carb count. That's why I specify blackstrap, the darkest, strongest molasses there is. It's nice to know that blackstrap is also where all the minerals they take out of sugar end up—it may be carby, but at least it's not a nutritional wasteland. Still, I only use small amounts. It's easiest to measure these small quantities if you store your blackstrap in a squeeze bottle—mine is in one of those plastic "honey bears."

You may be asking why I don't just use some of the artificial brown-sugar flavored sweeteners out there. The answer is because I've tried them, and I haven't tasted a one I would be willing to buy again. Ick.

Bouillon or broth concentrates. Bouillon or broth concentrate comes in cube, crystal, or liquid form. It is generally full of salt and chemicals and doesn't taste notably like the animal it supposedly came from. It definitely does *not* make a suitable substitute for good-quality broth if you're making a pot of soup. However, these products can be useful for adding a little kick of flavor here and there—more as seasonings than as soups—and for this use, I keep them on hand. I generally use chicken bouillon crystals because I find them easier to use than cubes. I also keep liquid beef broth concentrate on hand. I chose this because, unlike the cubes or crystals, it actually has a bit of beef in it. I use Wyler's, but I see no reason why any comparable product wouldn't work fine. If you can get the British product Bovril, it's probably even better!

Fish sauce. Called nuoc mam in Vietnam and nam pla in Thailand, this is a salty, fermented seasoning widely used in Southeast Asian cooking. It's available in Asian grocery stores and in the Asian foods section of big grocery stores. Grab it when you find it; it keeps nicely without refrigeration. Fish sauce is used in a few really great recipes in this book, and it adds an authentic flavor. In a pinch, you can substitute soy sauce, although you'll lose some of your Southeast Asian accent.

By the way, fish sauce is not the same thing as Chinese oyster sauce.

Guar and xanthan. These sound just dreadful, don't they? But they're in lots of your favorite processed foods, so how bad can they be? You're probably wondering what the heck they are, though. They're forms of water-soluble fiber, extracted and purified. Guar and xanthan are both flavorless white powders; their value to us is as low-carb thickeners. Technically speaking, these are carbs, but they're all fiber—nothing but. So don't worry about it.

Your health food store may well be able to order guar or xanthan for you—I slightly prefer xanthan, myself—if they don't have them on hand. You can also find suppliers online. Keep either one in a jar with a tight lid, and it will never go bad. I bought a pack of guar about 15 years ago and it's still going strong!

Low-carbohydrate bake mix. There are several brands of low-carbohydrate bake mix on the market. These are generally a combination of some form of powdery protein and/or fiber—soy, whey, sometimes oat—plus baking powder and sometimes salt. These are the low-carb world's equivalent of Bisquick, although low-carb bake mixes differ from Bisquick in that they do not have shortening added. You will need to add butter, oil, or some other form of fat when using these mixes to make pancakes, waffles, biscuits, and the like. I mostly use low-carb bake mix in lesser quantities for things like "flouring" chicken before baking or frying, or for making batter to fry onion rings in. If you can't find low-carbohydrate bake mix locally, there are many websites that sell it.

Bland oils. Sometimes you want to use a bland oil in a recipe—something that adds little or no flavor of its own. In this case, I recommend peanut, sunflower, or canola oil. These are the oils I mean when I simply say "oil." Avoid highly polyunsaturated oils such as safflower oil; they deteriorate quickly both from heat and from contact with oxygen, and they have been associated with an increased risk of cancer.

Olive oil. It surely will come as no surprise to you that olive oil is a healthy fat, but you may not know that there are various kinds. Extra-virgin olive oil is the first pressing. It is deep green, with a full, fruity flavor, and it makes all the difference in salad dressings. However, it is expensive and it's too strongly flavored for some uses. I keep a bottle of extra virgin olive oil on hand, but I use it exclusively for salads.

For sautéing and other general use, I use a grade of olive oil known as "pomace." Pomace is far cheaper than extra-virgin olive oil and has a milder flavor. I buy pomace in gallon cans at a local grocery specializing in Mediterranean foods. These gallon cans are worth looking for; it's the cheapest way to buy the stuff. If you can't find gallon cans of pomace, feel free to buy whatever cheaper, milder-flavored olive oil is available in your grocery store.

Be aware that if you refrigerate olive oil it will become solid. This is no big deal; it will be fine once it warms up again. If you need it quickly, you can run the bottle under warm water or microwave it for a minute or so on low power (assuming the container has no metal and will fit in your microwave).

Onions. Onions are a borderline vegetable; they're certainly higher in carbohydrates than, say, lettuce or cucumbers. However, they're loaded with valuable phytochemicals, so they're very healthful, and of course they add an unmatched flavor to all sorts of foods. Therefore I use onions a lot, but I try to use the least quantity that will give the desired flavor. Indeed, one of the most common things I do to cut carb counts on "borrowed" recipes is to cut back on the amount of onion used. If you have serious diabetes, you'll want to watch your quantities of onions pretty carefully and maybe even cut back further on the amounts I've given.

If you're not an accomplished cook, you need to know that different types of onions are good for different things. There are mild onions, which are best used raw, and there are stronger onions, which are what you want if you're going to be cooking with them. My favorite mild onions are sweet red onions; these are widely available, and you'll see that I've used them quite a lot in the recipes. However, if you prefer, you can substitute Vidalia or Bermuda onions anywhere I've specified sweet red onions. Scallions, also known as green onions, also are mild and are best eaten raw or quickly cooked in stir-fries. To me, scallions have their own flavor, and I generally don't substitute for them, but your kitchen won't blow up or anything if you use another sort of sweet onion in their place.

When a recipe simply says "onion," what I'm talking about is good old yellow globe onions, the ones you can buy in net sacks. You'll be doing yourself a favor if you pick a sack with smallish onions in it—that way, when a recipe calls for just 1/4 or 1/2 cup (30 to 50 g) of chopped onion, you're unlikely to be left with half an onion on your hands. For the record, when I say simply, "a small onion" I mean one about 1 1/2 inches (4 cm) in diameter, or about 1/4 to 1/3 cup (30 g) when chopped. A medium onion would be about 2 inches (5 cm) in diameter and would yield between 1/2 and 3/4 cup (50 and 75 g) when chopped. A large onion would be 2 1/2 to 3 inches (6 to 8 cm) across and will yield about 1 cup (115 g) when chopped. Personally, I'm not so obsessive about exact carb counts that I bother to measure every scrap of onion I put in a dish; I think in terms of small, medium, and large onions, instead. But that's up to you.

Packaged broths. Canned or boxed chicken broth and beef broth are very handy items to keep around, and they're certainly quicker than making your own. However, the quality of most of the canned broth you'll find at your local grocery store is appallingly bad. The chicken broth has all sorts of chemicals in it and often sugar, as well. The "beef" broth is worse—it frequently has no beef in it whatsoever. I refuse to use the majority of these products, and you should, too.

However, there are a few canned or boxed broths on the market worth buying. Many grocery stores now carry a brand called Kitchen Basics, which contains no chemicals at all. It is packaged in quart-size boxes (one litre in the UK), much like soy milk. Kitchen Basics comes in both chicken and beef. Health food stores also have good-quality canned and boxed broths—both Shelton and Health Valley brands are widely distributed in the United States.

Decent packaged broth will cost you a little more than the stuff that is made of salt and chemicals, but not a whole lot more. If you watch for sales, you can often get it as cheaply as the bad stuff, and stock up. When my health food store runs a sale on good broth, I buy piles of the stuff!

One last note—you will also find canned vegetable broth, particularly at health food stores. This is tasty, but it runs much higher in carbohydrates than the chicken and beef broths. I'd avoid it.

Rice protein powder. For use in savory recipes—entrées and such—you need protein powder that isn't sweet, and preferably one that has no flavor at all. There are a number of these on the market, and some are blander than others. I've tried several kinds, and I've found that rice protein powder is the one I like best. I buy Nutribiotic brand, which has 1 gram of carbohydrates per table-spoon, but any unflavored rice protein powder with a similar carb count should work fine. For that matter, I see no reason not to experiment with other unfla-vored protein powders, if you like. If you can't find rice protein powder, ask your local health food store to order it for you—most health food stores are lovely about special orders.

Splenda. Splenda is the latest artificial sweetener to hit the market, and it blows all of the competition clear out of the water! Feed nondieting friends and family Splenda-sweetened desserts and they will never know that you didn't use sugar. It tastes that good.

Splenda has some other advantages. The table sweetener has been bulked so that it measures spoon-for-spoon and cup-for-cup just like sugar. This makes adapting recipes much easier. Also, Splenda stands up to heat, unlike aspartame, which means you can use it in baked goods.

However, Splenda is *not* completely carb-free. Because of the malto-dextrin used to bulk it, Splenda has about 0.5 gram of carbohydrate per teaspoon, or about one eighth of the carbohydrates of sugar. So count 0.5 gram per teaspoon, 1 1/2 grams per tablespoon, and 24 grams per cup (100 g). At this writing, MacNeill, the company that makes Splenda, has no plans to release liquid Splenda in the United States, but I am hoping that they will change their minds. The liquid, available in some foreign countries, is carb-free, and while it will take a little more finesse to figure out quantities, it will allow me to slash the carb counts of all sorts of recipes still further.

Tomatoes and tomato products. Tomatoes are a borderline vegetable, but they are so nutritious, flavorful, and versatile that I'm reluctant to leave them out of low-carb cuisine entirely. After all, lycopene, the pigment that makes tomatoes red, has been shown to be a potent cancer-fighter. Who wants to miss out on something like that?

You'll notice that I call for canned tomatoes in a fair number of recipes, even some where fresh tomatoes might do. This is because fresh tomatoes aren't very good for much of the year, while canned tomatoes are all canned at the height of ripeness. I'd rather have a good canned tomato in my sauce or soup than a mediocre fresh one. Since canned tomatoes are generally used with all the liquid that's in the can, the nutritional content doesn't suffer the way it does with most canned vegetables.

Canned diced tomatoes with green chilies have become widely available in the past few years, and what a welcome addition they are! They let us add two great flavors by opening just one can.

I also use plain canned tomato sauce, canned pizza sauce, canned pasta sauce, and jarred salsa. When choosing these products, you need to be aware that tomatoes, for some reason, inspire food packers to flights of sugar-fancy. They add sugar, corn syrup, and other carb-laden sweeteners to all sorts of tomato products. So it is even more important that you read the labels on all tomato-based products to find the ones with no added sugar. And keep on reading them! The good, cheap brand of salsa I used for quite a while showed up one day with "New, Improved!" on the label. Guess how they'd improved it? Right. They'd added sugar. So I found a new brand.

Vege-Sal. If you've read my newsletter, *Lowcarbezine!*, you know that I'm a big fan of Vege-Sal. What is Vege-Sal? It's a salt that's been seasoned, but don't think "seasoned salt." Vege-Sal is much milder than traditional seasoned salt.

It's simply salt that's been blended with some dried, powdered vegetables. The flavor is quite subtle, but I think it improves all sorts of things. I've given you the choice between using regular salt or Vege-Sal in a wide variety of recipes. Don't worry, they'll all come out fine with plain old salt, but I do think Vege-Sal adds a little something extra. Vege-Sal is also excellent sprinkled over chops and steaks in place of regular salt. Vege-Sal is made by Modern Products and is widely available in health food stores.

Vinegar. Various recipes in this book call for wine vinegar, cider vinegar, rice vinegar, tarragon vinegar, white vinegar, and balsamic vinegar. If you've always thought that vinegar was just vinegar, think again! Each of these vinegars has a distinct flavor all its own, and if you substitute one for the other, you'll change the whole character of the recipe—one splash of cider vinegar in your Asian Chicken Salad, and you've traded your Chinese accent for an American twang. Vinegar is such a great way to give bright flavors to foods while adding few carbs that I keep all of these varieties on hand—it's not like they go bad or anything.

As with everything else, read the labels on your vinegar. I've seen cider vinegar that has 0 grams of carbohydrates per ounce, and I've seen cider vinegar that has 4 grams of carbohydrates per ounce—that's a huge difference! Beware, also, of apple cider *flavored* vinegar—white vinegar with artificial flavors added. I bought this once by mistake, so I thought I'd give you the heads-up. (You'd think the Label Reading Police would be beyond such errors, wouldn't you?)

Wine. There are several recipes in this cookbook calling for either dry red or dry white wine. I find the inexpensive wines that come in a mylar bag inside a cardboard box to be very convenient to keep on hand for cooking, for the simple reason that they do not go bad because the contents are never exposed to air. These are not fabulous vintage wines, but they're fine for our modest purposes, and they certainly are handy. I generally have both Burgundy and Chablis box wines on hand. Be wary of any wine with "added flavors"—too often, one of those flavors will be sugar. Buy wine with a recognizable name—Burgundy, Rhine, Chablis, Cabernet, and the like, rather than stuff like "Chillable Red."

chapter one

15~Minute Eggs

Actually, this is a misnomer—most of these egg dishes will take you well under 15 minutes!

Please, please don't think of eggs as being only for breakfast. Eggs are the ideal low-carb fast food at any time of day. They're cheap, they're tasty, they're nutritious, and they can be prepared in no time flat. With a carton of eggs in the refrigerator, you're never more than a few minutes away from a great meal!

We'll kick things off with omelets, the ultimate low-carb fast food. Once you know how to make an omelet, a whole world of fabulous, quick meals opens up to you.

Dana's Easy Omelet Method

You can learn this quickly. Really you can.

To start, you'll need a good pan. What's a "good pan"? I prefer a medium size skillet with a heavy bottom, sloping sides, and a nonstick surface. However, what I currently have is a 7-inch skillet with a heavy bottom, sloping sides, and a *formerly* nonstick surface. I can still make omelets in it, I just have to use a good shot of nonstick cooking spray. The heavy bottom and sloping sides, however, are essential.

Here's the really important thing to know about making omelets: The word "omelet" comes from a word meaning "to laminate," or to build up layers. And that's exactly what you do—you let a layer of beaten egg cook, then you lift up the edges and tip the pan so the raw egg runs under the cooked part. You do this all around the edges, of course, so you build it up evenly. The point is, you don't just let the beaten egg lie there in the skillet and wait for it to cook through; the bottom will be hopelessly overdone before the top is set.

So here's the start-to-finish omelet method:

1. First, have your filling ready. If you're using vegetables, you'll want to sauté them first. If you're using cheese, have it grated or sliced and ready to go. If you're making an omelet to use up leftovers (a great idea, by the way), warm them through in the microwave and have them standing by.

2. Spray your omelet pan well with nonstick spray if it doesn't have a good nonstick surface, and put it over high heat. While the skillet's heating, grab your eggs (2 is the perfect number for this size pan, but 1 or 3 will work, too) and a bowl, crack the eggs, and beat them with a fork. Don't add any water or milk or anything, just mix them up.

3. Test the heat of the pan. The pan is hot enough when a drop of water thrown in sizzles right away. Add a tablespoon of oil or butter, slosh it around to cover the bottom, then pour in the eggs, all at once. They should sizzle, too, and immediately start to set. When the bottom layer of egg is set around the edges—this should happen quite quickly—lift the edge using a spatula and tip the pan to let the raw egg flow underneath. Do this all around the edges, until there's not enough raw egg to run.

4. Now, turn your burner to the lowest heat if you have a gas stove. (If you have an electric stove, you'll have to have a "warm" burner standing by; electric elements don't cool off fast enough for this job.) Put your filling on one half of the omelet, cover the skillet, and let it sit over very low heat for a minute or two, no more. Peek and see if the raw, shiny egg is gone from the top surface (although you can serve it that way if you like; that's how the French prefer their omelets), and the cheese, if you've used it, is melted. If not, re-cover the skillet and let it sit for another minute or two.

5. When your omelet is done, slip a spatula under the half without the filling and fold it over, then lift the whole thing onto a plate. You could get fancy and tip the pan, letting the filling side of the omelet slide onto the plate and folding the top over as you go, but this takes some practice.

This makes a single-serving omelet. I think it's a lot easier to make several individual omelets than to make one big one, and omelets are so fast to make that it's not that big a deal to make more than one. Anyway, that way you can customize your omelets to each individual's taste. If you're making more than two or three omelets, keep them warm in your oven, set to its very lowest heat, until they're all ready to eat.

Now read on for some ideas for what to put in your omelets!

Omelets

☺ Apple, Bacon, and Blue Cheese Omelet

Three of my favorite things—wrapped in eggs, another of my favorite things!

> 3 slices bacon
>
> 1/4 Granny Smith or other crisp, tart apple, thinly sliced
>
> 2 teaspoons butter, divided
>
> 2 eggs, beaten
>
> 1 ounce crumbled blue cheese (30 g)

Start the bacon cooking in the microwave—if you don't own a microwave bacon rack, a glass pie plate will work just fine. (In my microwave, 3 to 4 minutes on High is about right, but microwave power varies.)

While the bacon's cooking, melt 1 teaspoon of butter in your omelet pan over medium-high heat. Add the apples, and fry for 2 to 3 minutes per side, or until they're slightly golden. Remove the apple slices and keep them on hand.

Melt the remaining butter in the skillet, slosh it about, and make your omelet according to Dana's Easy Omelet Method (see page 27), using nonstick cooking spray if necessary. Arrange the fried apples on half the omelet, top with the blue cheese, cover the pan, and turn the burner to low.

Go check on that bacon! If it needs another minute, do that now, while the cheese is melting. Then drain it and crumble it over the now-melted blue cheese. Fold and serve.

Yield: 1 serving, with 6 grams of carbohydrates and 1 gram of fiber, for a total of 5 grams of usable carbs and 23 grams of protein.

⏱ Chili Lime Pork Omelet

This is one of those omelets that makes it clear that eggs ain't just for breakfast anymore—this is definitely hearty enough for dinner. The Chili Lime Pork is very quick to make and keeps well in a closed container in the fridge.

> 2 eggs, beaten
>
> 1 to 2 teaspoons oil
>
> 1/4 batch Chili Lime Pork Strips (see page 114)
>
> 1/4 avocado, sliced
>
> 1/4 cup shredded Monterey Jack (30 g)
>
> Sour cream (optional)
>
> Salsa (optional)

Make your omelet according to Dana's Easy Omelet Method (see page 27). Arrange the Chili Lime Pork strips on half the omelet, and top with the avocado and the cheese. Cover, turn the burner to low, and let it cook for a minute or two to melt the cheese and finish setting the eggs. Fold and serve. Top with sour cream, salsa, or both if desired.

Yield: 1 serving, with 6 grams of carbohydrates and 2 grams of fiber, for a total of 4 grams of usable carbs and 42 grams of protein.

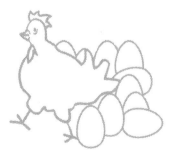

☺ "Clean the Fridge" Omelet

The name is not a joke—I made this omelet up out of whatever I found kicking around in the refrigerator, needing to be used up before it went bad. The results were definitely good enough to make it again.

> 1/2 red bell pepper, cut into thin strips
>
> 1/4 medium onion, thinly sliced
>
> 3 tablespoons olive oil
>
> 2 eggs, beaten
>
> 1 ounce jalapeño jack, shredded or sliced (30 g)
>
> 1/2 avocado, sliced

In your skillet over medium-high heat, sauté the pepper and onion in the oil until the onion is translucent and the pepper is going limp. Remove from the pan and keep on hand. If your pan isn't nonstick, give it a shot of nonstick cooking spray before putting it back on the burner and increasing the heat a touch to high. Make your omelet according to Dana's Easy Omelet Method (see page 27).
Put the cheese on half the omelet, top with the avocado and then the pepper and onion. Cover, turn the burner to low, and let it cook until the cheese is melted. Fold and serve.

Yield: 1 serving, with 14 grams of carbohydrates and 6 grams of fiber, for a total of 8 grams of usable carbs and 21 grams of protein.

❋ This also contains a whopping 821 milligrams of potassium!

⊕ Cumin Mushroom Omelet

Exotic and wonderful—and even if you're making the Cumin Mushrooms from scratch, you'll come in right around the 15-minute mark.

> 2 eggs, beaten
>
> 1 ounce Monterey Jack cheese, sliced or shredded (30 g)
>
> 1/3 batch Cumin Mushrooms (see page 192), warmed

Make your omelet according to Dana's Easy Omelet Method (see page 27). Put the cheese on half the omelet, then top with the mushrooms. Cover, turn the burner to low, and let it cook for 2 to 3 minutes, or until the cheese is melted. Fold and serve.

Yield: 1 serving, with 6 grams of carbohydrates and 1 gram of fiber, for a total of 5 grams of usable carbs and 20 grams of protein.

Variation: A couple of ounces (50 g) of purchased grilled chicken strips make a nice addition to this omelet. If you add the chicken, figure on 1 additional gram of carbohydrate (the chicken strips are marinated before cooking) and 6 additional grams of protein per ounce.

⊕ Caviar and Sour Cream Omelet

Caviar is one of those things—either you like it or you don't. If you do, why not eat it in an omelet? Sort of an "eggs meet eggs" thing.

> 2 eggs, beaten
>
> 1 tablespoon caviar
>
> 3 tablespoons sour cream

Make your omelet according to Dana's Easy Omelet Method (see page 27). Spread the caviar and sour cream over half the omelet. Cover, and turn the burner to low, and cook just another minute or so—you don't want your sour cream to "break." Fold and serve.

Yield: 1 serving, with 4 grams of carbohydrates, no fiber, and 16 grams of protein.

⏲ Curried Cheese and Olive Omelets

This was originally a spread for English muffins and the like, but it makes a wicked omelet. I know that this combination of ingredients sounds a little odd, but the flavor is magical.

> 1 cup shredded cheddar cheese (120 g)
>
> 5 or 6 scallions, finely sliced, including the crisp part of the green
>
> 4.25 ounce (120 g) can chopped ripe olives, drained
>
> 3 tablespoons mayonnaise
>
> 1/2 teaspoon curry powder
>
> 6 eggs, beaten

Simply plunk the cheese, scallions, olives, mayonnaise, and curry powder in a mixing bowl, and combine well. Now, make omelets according to Dana's Easy Omelet Method (see page 27), using the cheese-and-olive mixture as the filling. As the 6 eggs suggests, this makes 3 omelets. If there's only one of you, however, just use 2 eggs. The cheese mixture will keep well for a couple of days in a closed container in the refrigerator, letting you make fabulous omelets in far less than 15 minutes for a few days running.

Yield: 3 servings, each with 6 grams of carbohydrates and 3 grams of fiber, for a total of 3 grams of usable carbs and 21 grams of protein.

❈ As a bonus, you get 372 milligrams of calcium!

⊕ Tomato-Mozzarella Omelet

Sliced tomatoes and mozzarella are a time-honored Italian appetizer—and they make a great omelet filling, too.

>   2 eggs, beaten
>   1/3 cup shredded mozzarella (50 g)
>   1/2 small tomato, sliced
>   2 tablespoons chopped fresh basil

Make your omelet according to Dana's Easy Omelet Method (see page 27). Cover half the omelet with the cheese, then top with the tomato slices. Cover, turn the burner to low, and let it cook for 2 to 3 minutes, or until the cheese is melted. Scatter the basil over the filling, fold, and serve.

Yield: 1 serving, with 5 grams of carbohydrates and 1 gram of fiber, for a total of 4 grams of usable carbs and 20 grams of protein.

✳ You'll also get 296 milligrams of potassium and 272 milligrams of calcium.

⊕ Curried Tuna Omelets

These taste really different and really good!

>   2 eggs, beaten
>   1/3 batch Curried Tuna Salad (see page 122)

Make your omelet according to Dana's Easy Omelet Method (see page 27). Cover half the omelet with the tuna salad. Cover, turn the burner to low, and cook long enough to warm through. Fold and serve.

Yield: 1 serving, with 7 grams of carbohydrates and 2 grams of fiber, for a total of 5 grams of usable carbs and 33 grams of protein.

☉ Kasseri Tapenade Omelet

Cool Greek flavors! Look for jars of tapenade, an olive relish, in big grocery stores. Kasseri is a Greek cheese; all my local grocery stores carry it, so I'm guessing yours do, too.

> 2 to 3 teaspoons olive oil
>
> 2 eggs, beaten
>
> 1 ounce kasseri cheese, sliced or shredded (30 g)
>
> 1 1/2 tablespoons tapenade

Make your omelet according to Dana's Easy Omelet Method (see page 27). Cover half the omelet with the cheese, and then top with the tapenade. Cover, turn the burner to low, and let it cook for a couple of minutes, until the cheese is melted. Fold and serve.

Yield: 1 serving, with 4 grams of carbohydrates, no fiber, and 18 grams of protein.

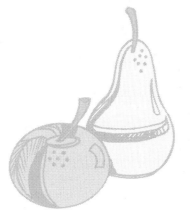

Scrambles

Think of scrambles as omelets for the faint of heart. And please, feel free to experiment with scrambles of your own! The variety of things that taste good when added to scrambled eggs is never-ending.

☺ Smoked Salmon and Goat Cheese Scramble

Sounds fancy, I know, but this takes almost no time and is very impressive. It's terrific to make for a special brunch or a late-night supper. A simple green salad with a classic vinaigrette dressing would be perfect with this.

> 4 eggs
> 1/2 cup heavy cream (120 ml)
> 1 teaspoon dried dill weed
> 4 scallions
> 1/4 pound chevre (goat cheese) (125 g)
> 1/4 pound moist smoked salmon (125 g)
> 1 to 2 tablespoons butter

Whisk the eggs together with the cream and dill weed. Slice the scallions thin, including the crisp part of the green. Cut the chevre—it will have a texture similar to cream cheese—into little hunks. Coarsely crumble the smoked salmon.

In a big (preferably nonstick) skillet, melt the butter over medium-high heat. (If your skillet doesn't have a nonstick surface, give it a shot of nonstick cooking spray before adding the butter.) When the butter's melted, add the scallions first, and sauté them for just a minute. Add the eggs and cook, stirring frequently, until they're halfway set—about 1 minute to 90 seconds. Add the chevre and smoked salmon, continue cooking and stirring until the eggs are set, and serve.

Yield: 3 servings, each with 5 grams of carbohydrates and 1 gram of fiber, for a total of 4 grams of usable carbs and 27 grams of protein.

☻ Deviled Ham and Eggs

If you don't have leftover ham lying around the house, you can buy modest-size chunks of pre-cooked ham in any grocery store. Useful stuff!

> ½ tablespoon butter
>
> ½ cup smallish ham cubes (50 g)
>
> ¼ cup chopped onion (30 g)
>
> 3 eggs
>
> 1 teaspoon spicy brown or Dijon mustard
>
> 1 teaspoon prepared horseradish

Melt the butter in a small skillet over medium heat. Add the ham and onion, and sauté until the onion is translucent and the ham has a touch of gold. Scramble the eggs with the mustard and horseradish, and pour them over the ham and onion in the skillet. Scramble until the eggs are set, and serve.

Yield: 1 serving, with 8 grams of carbohydrates (less if you use really low-carb ham) and 1 gram of fiber, for a total of 7 grams of usable carbs and 29 grams of protein.

⊕ Parmesan Rosemary Eggs

This is so simple and so wonderful. If you like Italian food, you have to try this. It's also easy to double or triple.

> 3 eggs
> 2 tablespoons heavy cream
> 1/4 cup grated Parmesan cheese (30 g)
> 1/2 teaspoon ground rosemary*
> 1/2 teaspoon minced garlic
> 1/2 tablespoon butter

* You can use whole, dried rosemary, but you'll have little needles in your food. If you do use whole rosemary, increase the amount to 1 teaspoon.

Whisk together the eggs, cream, cheese, rosemary, and garlic. Put a medium-size skillet over medium-high heat (if it isn't nonstick, give it a shot of nonstick cooking spray first). When the pan is hot, add the butter, give the egg mixture one last stir to make sure the cheese hasn't settled to the bottom, then pour the egg mixture into the skillet. Scramble until the eggs are set, and serve.

Yield: 1 serving, with 3 grams of carbohydrates, a trace of fiber, and 25 grams of protein.

⊕ Blue Eggs

Wow—scrambled eggs with blue cheese and herbs. Yum!

> 4 eggs
> 2 tablespoons crumbled blue cheese
> 3 scallions, finely sliced
> 2 tablespoons chopped parsley
> 1/8 teaspoon dried marjoram
> 1/8 teaspoon dried thyme

Just scramble up the eggs, add the cheese, scallions, parsley, marjoram, and thyme, and stir it all up. Give your big, heavy skillet a shot of nonstick cooking spray, heat it over medium-high heat, and pour in the egg and cheese mixture. Scramble until set, and serve.

Yield: 1 or 2 servings. Assuming 2 servings, each will have 3 grams of carbohydrates and 1 gram of fiber, for a total of 2 grams of usable carbs and 13 grams of protein.

☉ Moroccan Scramble

With all these vegetables, this is a meal in itself. Exotic and fabulous.

> 1 tablespoon olive oil
>
> 1/4 cup chopped onion (30 g)
>
> 1/2 teaspoon minced garlic or 1 clove garlic, crushed
>
> 1 tablespoon tapenade
>
> 1/4 cup canned diced tomatoes (50 ml)
>
> 3 eggs
>
> 1/2 teaspoon ground cumin
>
> 2 tablespoons chopped fresh cilantro
>
> Salt and pepper

In a skillet, heat the olive oil over high heat, and start sautéing the onion and garlic. When the onion is translucent, add the tapenade and tomatoes, and stir. Now, whisk the eggs with the cumin, and pour the eggs into the vegetable mixture. Scramble until mostly set, then add the cilantro and scramble until done. Salt and pepper to taste, and serve.

Yield: 1 serving, with 11 grams of carbohydrates and 1 gram of fiber, for a total of 10 grams of usable carbs and 18 grams of protein.

⏱ French Country Scramble

This is for anyone who doesn't think that eggs can be elegant.

> 4 ounces sliced mushrooms (120 g)
>
> 3 scallions, coarsely sliced
>
> 1 tablespoon butter
>
> 2 canned artichoke hearts, chopped
>
> 6 eggs
>
> 1/2 cup shredded Gruyère (120 g)

If you haven't purchased your mushrooms already sliced, slice 'em up while you slice the scallions. In a large, heavy skillet over medium-high heat, sauté the mushrooms and scallions in the butter. When the mushrooms have turned darker, add the artichoke hearts (I just slice mine right into the skillet), and stir the whole thing up. Then beat the eggs, add them to the skillet, and scramble the whole thing. When the eggs are about half-set, add the cheese, and scramble until done. Serve.

Yield: 2 or 3 servings. Assuming 3 servings, each will have 10 grams of carbohydrates and 4 grams of fiber, for a total of 6 grams of usable carbs and 19 grams of protein. Note: Keep in mind that much of the carbohydrate in artichokes is in the form of inulin, about the lowest-impact carbohydrate yet discovered, so the blood sugar impact is less than the numbers would imply—which is pretty low to begin with.

☺ Huevos Con El Sabor de Chiles Rellenos

Chiles Rellenos—green chilies stuffed with cheese, dipped in batter, and then fried—are irresistible, and very time-consuming to make. However, since the traditional batter is egg-rich, it occurred to me to incorporate the chilies and the cheese into a scramble. It's delicious! If you haven't tried canned green chilies, you should know that they're only slightly spicy—this recipe won't leave you gasping and reaching for a glass of water.

> 6 eggs
>
> 1/4 cup canned diced green chilies (30 g)
>
> 1 tablespoon butter or oil
>
> 4 ounces Monterey Jack cheese, cut into small chunks (100 g)

Beat the eggs with the chilies. Spray a large, heavy skillet with nonstick cooking spray, and put it over medium-high heat. When the skillet is hot, add the butter or oil, and slosh it around to coat the bottom of the skillet.

Pour in the beaten eggs with chilies, and scramble them until they're about half-set. Add the chunks of Monterey Jack, continue scrambling until set, then serve.

Yield: 2 or 3 servings. Assuming 2 servings, each will have 4 grams of carbohydrates, a trace of fiber, and 31 grams of protein.

☺ Hangtown Fry

This is a very famous dish originating, I believe, in the Gold Rush days of California.

> 8 large oysters
>
> 2 tablespoons low-carb bake mix or 2 tablespoons rice protein powder
>
> 4 tablespoons butter
>
> 4 eggs
>
> 2 tablespoons cream
>
> 2 tablespoons grated Parmesan cheese
>
> 2 tablespoons chopped parsley

Coat the oysters with the bake mix or protein powder, either by putting the bake mix or protein powder in a shallow dish and rolling the oysters in it or by shaking them in a small brown paper bag with the mix in it.

Melt the butter over medium heat in a large, heavy skillet. Add the oysters, and fry until golden all over, about 5 to 7 minutes.

While the oysters are frying, beat the eggs and the cream together. When the oysters are golden, pour the beaten eggs into the skillet, and scramble until set. Divide between 2 serving plates, sprinkle a tablespoon of Parmesan and a tablespoon of parsley over each portion, and serve.

Yield: 2 servings, each with 5 grams of carbohydrates and 1 gram of fiber, for a total of 4 grams of usable carbs and 21 grams of protein.

☉ Cottage Egg Scramble

Eggs scrambled with cottage cheese are surprisingly good, and of course the cottage cheese adds nutrients the eggs lack—most notably calcium. With a salad on the side, this is a great simple supper for a tired night.

4 eggs

1/2 cup small-curd cottage cheese (120 g)

1/8 teaspoon dried basil

1/2 green pepper, finely chopped

1 tablespoon butter

1/4 cup shredded cheddar cheese (30 g)

Beat the eggs and cottage cheese together, and stir in the basil. In a large, heavy skillet over medium-high heat, sauté the green pepper in the butter (you might want to give that skillet a shot of nonstick cooking spray first). When the pepper is getting a little soft, add the egg mixture and scramble. When the eggs are almost set, add the cheddar, and continue scrambling until the eggs are completely set. Serve.

Yield: 2 servings, each with 5 grams of carbohydrates and 1 gram of fiber, for a total of 4 grams of usable carbs and 23 grams of protein.

⊕ Chipotle Eggs

Smoky and complex, chipotle peppers—smoked jalapeños—are very special, and they make these eggs very special, too. Personally, I think a side of avocado slices with a little lime or lemon juice would be nice with this.

> ½ cup finely chopped onion (50 g)
>
> ½ teaspoon minced garlic or 1 clove garlic, crushed
>
> 1 tablespoon oil
>
> 2 small chipotle peppers canned in adobo sauce, finely minced—about 2 teaspoons
>
> 6 eggs
>
> ½ cup shredded Monterey Jack cheese (50 g)

Spray a large, heavy skillet with nonstick cooking spray, place it over medium-high heat, and start sautéing the onion and garlic in the oil. When the onion is translucent, add the chopped chipotles, stir them in, and let the whole thing cook for another minute. (This is a good time to break and scramble the eggs.)

Pour the eggs into the skillet and scramble until nearly set. Scatter the cheese evenly over the top, turn the burner to low, cover the skillet, and let it keep cooking until the cheese is melted—just a minute or two. Serve.

Yield: 2 or 3 servings. Assuming 2 servings, each will have 5 grams of carbohydrates and 1 gram of fiber, for a total of 4 grams of usable carbs and 24 grams of protein.

✵ This also contains 285 milligrams of calcium and 248 milligrams of potassium. (More potassium if you have those avocado slices!)

⊕ Houbyfest Eggs

"What the heck is 'Houbyfest'?" I hear you cry. "Houby" is Czech for "mushroom," and Houbyfest is an annual mushroom celebration in the heavily Bohemian Chicago suburb of Berwyn. This dish is so loaded with mushrooms—as much mushroom as egg—that the name seemed appropriate.

8 ounces sliced mushrooms (250 g)

2 tablespoons butter

1 teaspoon dried thyme

1/2 teaspoon minced garlic or 1 clove garlic, crushed

2 scallions, sliced

6 eggs

2 tablespoons chopped fresh parsley (optional)

In a large, heavy skillet, sauté the mushrooms in the butter over medium-high heat. When the mushrooms have turned dark, stir in the thyme, garlic, and scallions, and let them cook for a minute or two while you crack and scramble the eggs. Then pour the eggs into the skillet, scramble, and serve.
A little fresh parsley scattered over this is nice, but not essential.

Yield: 2 or 3 servings. Assuming 2 servings, each will have 9 grams of carbohydrates and 2 grams of fiber, for a total of 7 grams of usable carbs and 19 grams of protein.

✵ This dish has 633 milligrams potassium!

☺ Eggs Fu Yong

This can be made on the stove top, is quick and cheap to make, uses up any sort of leftover meat, is high in protein and low in carbohydrates, needs no side dishes, is infinitely variable, and tastes good, to boot! How much more can you ask from a recipe? Because this recipe can be varied so much, what I've given you is more a guideline than hard and fast rules.

4 eggs

2 teaspoons dry sherry

1 tablespoon soy sauce

Peanut oil, or other bland oil for frying

1/2 teaspoon grated gingerroot

2 to 3 ounces leftover cooked meat, cut into small strips* (50-90 g)
   or 2 to 3 ounces canned chunk turkey, chicken, or ham, or canned shrimp
   or crabmeat (50-90 g)

1 cup Napa cabbage or green cabbage, finely shredded, or bagged coleslaw
   mix (75 g), or 1 cup bean sprouts (50 g), or some combination of the two

1/4 cup mushrooms, canned or fresh, finely chopped (30 g)

1/4 cup onion or scallions, finely minced (30 g)

1/4 cup bamboo shoots, cut into matchstick strips (30 g)

* Use ham, pork, turkey, chicken, or shrimp—whatever you've got. If they're little bitty shrimp, leave 'em whole. If they're great big shrimp, chop them coarsely.

Beat the eggs with the sherry and the soy sauce. Set aside. In a large skillet, heat a few tablespoons of oil over high heat. Add the ginger, then the meat and vegetables. Stir-fry until the onion is translucent and the cabbage or bean sprouts are tender-crisp. Stir the meat and vegetables into the seasoned eggs. Add another few tablespoons of oil to the skillet, and heat.

Ladle in about 1/2 cup (120 ml) of the egg mixture at a time, and fry on both sides until the egg is set.

You can cook this in a wok if you want to be terribly authentic, but I actually find that a skillet is a lot easier for this recipe.

Yield: 2 servings. The carb count will vary a little, but each serving will have close to 6 grams of carbohydrates and 2 grams of fiber, for a total of 4 grams of usable carbs and 26 grams of protein.

⏱ Asparagi All'Uovo

This Italian dish turns a couple of eggs into a light supper. This looks like a lot of instructions, but none of the steps takes much time.

>   1 pound asparagus (500 g)
>   ¼ cup olive oil (50 ml)
>   ½ teaspoon minced garlic or 1 clove garlic, crushed
>   ½ cup grated Parmesan cheese (75 g)
>   8 eggs

Start by snapping the bottoms off the asparagus where they break naturally. Put the asparagus in a microwaveable casserole or a glass pie plate. Add a couple of tablespoons of water, and cover. (Use plastic wrap or a plate to cover a pie plate.) Microwave on High for 3 to 4 minutes.

While the asparagus is cooking, stir the garlic into the olive oil.

When the asparagus is done, drain it. If you have 4 single-serving oven-proof dishes long enough to hold asparagus, they're ideal for this recipe—divide the asparagus between the 4 dishes. If not, you'll need to use a rectangular glass baking dish. Arrange the asparagus in 4 groups in the baking dish.

Whether you're using the individual dishes or the single baking dish, drizzle each serving of asparagus with the garlic and olive oil. Salt and pepper lightly, and divide the cheese between the 4 servings. Put the asparagus under the broiler, about 4 inches (10 cm) from low heat. Let it broil for 4 to 5 minutes.

While the asparagus is broiling, fry the eggs to your liking. Either use your biggest skillet to do them all at once, or divide them between two skillets.

When the Parmesan is lightly golden, take the asparagus out of the broiler. If you've cooked it in one baking dish, use a big spatula to carefully transfer each serving of asparagus to a plate. Top each serving of asparagus with 2 fried eggs, and serve.

Yield: 4 servings, each with 4 grams of carbohydrates and 1 gram of fiber, for a total of 3 grams of usable carbs and 16 grams of protein. If you'd like 22 grams of protein, add a third egg to each serving.

⏱ Blintzlets

This falls somewhere between a blintz and an omelet—hence the name. These are not dirt-low in carbs, but they're really yummy. They can be a special breakfast—you'll want to add a little more protein on the side, maybe some ham—or even a light dessert.

> 1 cup cottage cheese* (225 g)
>
> 2 tablespoons sour cream
>
> 1/2 teaspoon vanilla extract
>
> 1 tablespoon Splenda
>
> 4 eggs
>
> 1/4 cup vanilla whey protein powder (30 g)
>
> 6 tablespoons low-sugar strawberry preserves

* I use 4% fat cottage cheese; don't drop below 2%.

Put the cottage cheese, sour cream, vanilla, and Splenda in your food processor with the S-blade in place. Process until smooth.

Put the eggs and the protein powder in a blender, and whirl for 20 seconds or so.

Heat an 8- or 9-inch (2- or 25 cm) nonstick skillet over medium-high heat. Make sure it's hot before you cook! Even though it's nonstick, spray it with nonstick cooking spray. Now, pour in a small puddle of the egg mixture, and swirl the pan to coat the whole bottom—the idea is to use just enough of the egg mixture to cover the bottom of the skillet with a thin but solid layer. Cook until the top of the egg is set—this takes only a minute or so—then turn briefly. The protein powder makes this mixture very fragile, so be careful.

Lay the thin, eggy pancake on a plate, spread 1 tablespoon of the preserves on one half, and spoon 3 tablespoons of the cottage cheese mixture over it. Fold and serve. Repeat.

Yield: Makes 6, each with 9 grams of carbohydrates and 11 grams of protein. You can cut the carb count of each serving 3 grams by using just 1/2 tablespoon of preserves in each one. Or you could thaw 1/2 cup (150 g) of frozen unsweetened strawberries, mash them with a tablespoon or two of Splenda, and use them in place of the preserves. This would save 5 grams of carbs per serving—but you'll be pushing that 15-minute time limit.

⏲ Vedgeree

Kedgeree is a traditional dish made with rice; flaked, smoked mackerel or halibut; and hard-boiled eggs. I wanted to decarb it, but smoked mackerel and halibut are hard to come by, and I refuse to include impossible-to-find ingredients. Then I found a recipe for "Vedgeree," a vegetarian take-off, so I decarbed it, and it was yummy. This recipe will make a satisfying one-dish meal out of a couple of hard-boiled eggs. You do keep hard-boiled eggs in the fridge, don't you?

1/4 head cauliflower

1/2 cup frozen cross-cut green beans (75 g)

1/4 cup chopped onion (30 g)

1 cup sliced mushrooms (100 g)

1/2 tablespoon butter

2 hard-boiled eggs

Salt and pepper

Run the cauliflower through the shredding blade of a food processor. Put the cauliflower in a microwaveable dish, put the frozen green beans on top, add a couple of tablespoons of water, cover, and microwave on High for 7 minutes.

While the cauliflower and beans are cooking, sauté the onion and mushrooms in the butter until the onions are limp and translucent and the mushrooms have turned dark. Peel the eggs, quarter them lengthwise, and set them aside.

When the cauliflower and beans are done, pull them out, drain them, and stir them into the mushrooms and onions. Salt and pepper to taste. Place the hard-boiled egg quarters on top of the vegetables, turn the burner to low, cover the pan, and let the whole thing cook for just another minute or two, to heat the eggs through. Serve.

Yield: 1 serving, with 14 grams of carbohydrates and 4 grams of fiber, for a total of 10 grams of usable carbs and 16 grams of protein.

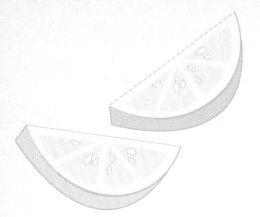

chapter two

15-Minute Tortilla Tricks

Yes, there are low-carbohydrate tortillas! They're made by La Tortilla Factory, and they're loaded with fiber, which is why they're low carb—each tortilla has 12 grams of carbohydrate and 9 grams of fiber, for a total of just 3 grams of usable carbs.

As the popularity of low-carb dieting has increased, these low-carb tortillas have become easier to find in stores—I know a couple of places that carry them here in Bloomington, Indiana, and it's not like we're the retail capital of the universe. Look around. If you can't find them, consider asking a local health food store to special order them for you—most health food stores are really helpful about special orders, and if enough people ask for the tortillas, the store may start carrying them as a matter of course.

If even that fails, go online and do a search for "low-carbohydrate tortillas." You'll find dozens of e-tailers happy to ship them to you.

I keep my low-carb tortillas in the freezer because I tend not to eat them up before they go stale or moldy. I've found it's a good idea to put a paper towel between each tortilla before freezing them. This keeps them from sticking together and also keeps them from getting soggy as they thaw (I also break off any obvious frost before thawing). Speaking of thawing, the tortillas thaw quite quickly, being so thin and all, but you can speed up the process by giving them a minute or so on low power—20 to 30 percent—in the microwave.

Low-carb tortillas are not exactly like either flour or corn tortillas; they have a flavor and texture of their own. We really enjoy them, and they sure are versatile! With a package of low-carb tortillas in the house and some cheese in the fridge, you've got a quick meal, any time.

I have tried making low-carb tortilla chips by cutting low-carb tortillas into wedges and frying them. The results were edible, but not great—tough, and a bit cardboardy. Feel free to try it if you'd like. Me, I'd rather have nuts or fiber crackers or something.

Since I didn't like the low-carb tortilla chips, I haven't tried frying these low-carb tortillas to make taco shells or tostadas. I think the low-carb tortillas are best left in their original soft-and-pliable state. This chapter will teach you a few ways to use them.

◷ Quesadillas

Is there anyone left who hasn't tried this Mexican version of the grilled cheese sandwich? If you'd like to make a single-serving quesadilla, use a single tortilla, cover half of it with cheese, and fold it over. Heck, you can use this method for all your quesadillas if you like; I just find the sandwiching method easier.

> 2 low-carb tortillas
> 4 ounces cheese, sliced or shredded (120 g)*

* Mexican Queso Quesadilla is the classic choice, but Monterey Jack, jalapeño jack, and cheddar are all great, too.

Put one tortilla in the bottom of a large, heavy, dry skillet over medium heat. Spread the cheese over it, and place the other tortilla on top. Let it cook a few minutes, until the cheese is starting to melt. Carefully flip the whole thing, and let it cook on the other side until the cheese is well-melted. Remove from the skillet, cut the quesadilla into quarters—a pizza cutter works well—and serve.

Yield: 2 servings, each with 12 grams of carbohydrates and 9 grams of fiber, for a total of 3 grams of usable carbs and 19 grams of protein.

❋ Each serving also contains 463 milligrams of calcium!

☉ Mondo Giganto Quesadilla-from-Hell

Zowie—this is a serious meal. Thank my husband for the name—he took one look at this big, thick quesadilla, and that's what he called it.

> 2 low-carb tortillas
>
> 3 ounces shredded Monterey Jack (90 g)
>
> 3 ounces purchased grilled chicken strips (90 g)
>
> 1/2 tablespoon canned sliced jalapeños
>
> 1/4 ripe avocado, sliced

Place one of the tortillas in a large, heavy, dry skillet. Spread half the shredded cheese on it, then top with the chicken, jalapeños, and avocado slices, and top with the rest of the cheese. Place the second tortilla on top. Toast over medium heat, with a tilted lid, for 3 to 4 minutes, or until the cheese is melting. Flip your Quesadilla-From-Hell carefully—a few bits may escape from the sides because it's so full of yumminess; just tuck the bits back in. Continue toasting until all the cheese is melted. I find it easiest to use a pizza cutter to cut this in quarters right in the pan (turn the heat off first). The quarters are far easier to transfer to plates than the whole bursting-at-the-seams thing.

Yield: 2 servings, each with 14 grams of carbohydrates and 10 grams of fiber, for a total of 4 grams of usable carbs and 29 grams of protein.

Tip: If you don't have purchased grilled chicken strips in the house, you can, of course, just throw a boneless, skinless chicken breast in your electric tabletop grill for 5 to 6 minutes, and then slice it up. This is good without the chicken, too, although lower in protein, of course. (The carb count drops 1 gram for each ounce of chicken)

⊕ Tortilla Pizza

This makes a great snack or light lunch. Keep in mind that the sauce is the highest carb part of this; don't go increasing the quantity.

> 1 low-carb tortilla
>
> 1 1/2 tablespoons no-sugar-added pizza sauce
>
> 1/2 cup shredded mozzarella cheese (50 g)

Place the tortilla on the baking tray of the toaster oven. Spread the pizza sauce over it, then top with the cheese. Bake in the toaster oven at 450°F (230°C, Gas Mark 8) until the cheese is bubbly and starting to brown (about 5 minutes). Cut into wedges and devour, watching out for pizza burns!

If you don't have a toaster oven, you have a couple of options: You can make the pizza in a conventional oven, but it will take a while to get up to 450°F (230°C, Gas Mark 8). You can cook it in a dry skillet, like an open-faced quesadilla—but you won't flip it, of course! This will melt the cheese, especially if you cover the pan with a tilted lid, but the cheese won't brown. If I were doing it this way, I'd cook it until the cheese was just melting, then put the whole skillet under the broiler for a minute to brown the cheese. (Make sure your skillet has an oven-proof handle, if you decide to do this.) Or you could just put the pizza sauce and cheese on half of the tortilla and fold it over like a quesadilla.

Yield: 1 serving, with 16 grams of carbohydrates and 9 grams of fiber, for a total of 7 grams of usable carbs (you can drop it a little lower by using really low-carb pizza sauce) and 18 grams of protein.

Note: Ragu makes a good pizza sauce with no added sugar that's widely available. However, they also make one with sugar (corn syrup, actually), so read the label!

⏱ Not-Just-for-Breakfast Burrito

I know most people won't do this much cooking when they're trying to get out of the house in the morning. However, this makes a killer lunch or supper, or even a hefty snack—and if you do want a really solid, incredibly yummy breakfast, be aware that I had this not only made but eaten well inside the 15-minute mark!

> 1 low-carb tortilla
>
> 2 ounces shredded Monterey Jack cheese (50 g)
>
> 2 scallions
>
> ¼ ripe avocado
>
> 2 eggs
>
> 2 tablespoons salsa
>
> 1 tablespoon sour cream
>
> 1 tablespoon chopped cilantro (optional, but mighty tasty)

Place the tortilla on a plate, and spread the cheese over it. Place the plate in your microwave. Don't nuke it yet, though.

Slice the scallions, and peel and slice the avocado.

Spray a medium-size skillet with nonstick cooking spray and put it over medium-high heat. Now take a second to go set your microwave for 60 seconds at 50 percent power. Start the microwave, come back, beat the eggs, pour them into the skillet, and scramble them until they're set. Turn off the heat under the pan.

Pull the tortilla with its melted cheese out of the microwave. Arrange the scrambled eggs down the middle, then top with the scallions, avocado, salsa, sour cream, and cilantro if you have some in the house. Fold as best you can—the burrito will be full to bursting!—and eat with the help of several napkins. Unbelievable!

Yield: 1 serving, with 22 grams of carbohydrates and 13 grams of fiber, for a total of 9 grams of usable carbs and 33 grams of protein.

✻ This burrito also packs 680 milligrams of potassium and 582 milligrams of calcium!

chapter three

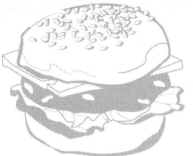

15~Minute Burgers

When we first discussed this project, my editor, Holly, and I discussed recipes that simply wouldn't work for the 15-minute framework. Holly brought up meat loaves. "Hah!" I said. "I'll just make them as burgers."

And that's what I've done. Here, for your quick-cooking, low-carbing pleasure, is an astonishing variety of interesting burger recipes, not a few of which originated as high-carb meat loaf recipes.

All of these recipes assume that you have an electric tabletop grill—you know, the George Foreman kind of thing. Since these grills cook from both sides, they cook very rapidly. If you don't have one, no worries—there's no reason you can't cook these burgers in a skillet, or even broil them—it'll just take an extra 5 minutes or so, and you'll have to flip them.

By the way, you'll find a number of burger recipes here that use pork. If you don't eat pork, I don't see any reason why ground turkey wouldn't work in these recipes. It would taste different, but should still taste good. If you do this, chop all of your other ingredients in a food processor, then add the ground turkey and pulse just long enough to combine.

☺ Beef, Sausage, and Spinach Burgers

These are superb, and of course they have enough vegetables in them that you don't really have to eat anything else with them if you don't want to take the trouble—but some bagged Italian salad mix with Italian or Creamy Garlic dressing would sure go well!

1 pound ground beef (500 g)

1/2 pound Italian sausage, hot or mild (225 g)

10-ounce package chopped frozen spinach, thawed (300 g)

1 teaspoon minced garlic or 2 cloves garlic, crushed

2 teaspoons Italian seasoning

1/2 teaspoon red pepper flakes

2 tablespoons oat bran

1 egg

3 tablespoons grated Parmesan cheese

1/2 teaspoon salt

1/2 cup no-sugar-added spaghetti sauce (125 ml)

2 tablespoons sliced ripe olives

Extra Parmesan for topping

Preheat your electric tabletop grill.

Dump the ground beef, sausage, spinach, garlic, seasoning, red pepper, oat bran, egg, cheese, and salt into a big bowl. (If your Italian sausage came in casings—mine did—slit them and squeeze out the meat, discarding the casings.) Using clean hands, smoosh everything together very well; you want the flavors of the two meats completely blended.

Form into 5 burgers, each about 1 inch (2 cm) thick. Slap 'em on the electric grill and set a timer for 6 minutes.

While the burgers are cooking, combine the spaghetti sauce and olives in a microwaveable bowl, and nuke for 1 minute at 70 percent power.

When the stove timer goes off, stick a burger with a fork. If the juices run clear, they're done. If they're pink, give the burgers another minute. When they're cooked through, transfer them to serving plates, top each with the spaghetti sauce and olives, plus more Parmesan if you like, and serve.

Yield: 5 servings, each with 9 grams of carbohydrates and 3 grams of fiber, for a total of 6 grams of usable carbs and 26 grams of protein, not counting any extra Parmesan you may put on top.

❀ This recipe's a good source of calcium and vitamin A, too!

☉ Apple Sausage Burgers

Feel free to make these with turkey sausage, if you prefer.

> ½ medium onion, peeled and cut in a few chunks
> ½ Granny Smith or other crisp, tart apple, cut into a few chunks (no need to peel it)
> 1 ½ pounds bulk pork sausage, hot or mild (750 g)
> 1 teaspoon dried thyme
> 1 teaspoon dried sage
> 1 teaspoon pepper

Preheat your electric tabletop grill.

Put the onion and apple in a food processor with the S-blade in place, and pulse until they're chopped to a medium consistency. Add the sausage, thyme, sage, and pepper, and pulse until it's all well-blended.

Form into 4 burgers, and put them on the grill. Cook for 7 minutes, or until the juices run clear.

Yield: 4 servings, each with 7 grams of carbohydrates and 1 gram of fiber, for a total of 6 grams of usable carbs and 20 grams of protein.

☉ Apple Cheddar Pork Burgers

What can I say? I think apples and pork are a terrific combination.

1/2 Granny Smith or other crisp, tart apple, cut into a few chunks
   (no need to peel it)

1/4 medium onion, peeled and cut into a couple of chunks

1 pound boneless pork loin, cut into 1 1/2-inch (4 cm) cubes (500 g)

2 tablespoons oat bran

1 egg

1/2 teaspoon salt or Vege-Sal

2 teaspoons prepared horseradish

2 ounces cheddar cheese, shredded (50 g)

Preheat your electric tabletop grill.

Put the apple, onion, pork, oat bran, egg, salt, and horseradish in a food processor, and pulse until the meat is ground and everything is well-blended. Add the cheese, and pulse just long enough to blend it in—we're trying to keep some actual shreds of cheese, here.

Form into 4 burgers, and slap 'em on the grill. Cook for 7 minutes, or until the juices run clear.

Yield: 4 servings, each with 5 grams of carbohydrates and 1 gram of fiber, for a total of 4 grams of usable carbs and 25 grams of protein.

☻ Cranberry Burgers

Someone anonymously posted a recipe for burgers with cranberry jelly in them to the Internet. It was clearly high-carb, but it looked so tasty that I had to figure out a way to adapt it. Here it is! Don't panic at this list of ingredients because this really is quite quick and easy—you just dump stuff in the food processor and run it.

5 slices bacon

1 small onion, peeled and cut into chunks

1/3 cup whole cranberries (30 g)

2 cloves fresh garlic or 1 teaspoon minced garlic

1/4 green pepper, core and seeds removed, cut into a couple of chunks

1 stalk celery, cut into a few chunks

1 pound ground beef (500 g)

2 tablespoons oat bran (30 ml)

1 egg

1/4 cup Splenda (30 g)

1/2 teaspoon grated gingerroot

5 ounces cheddar cheese, in slices (150 g)

First, begin cooking the bacon in the microwave, using either a microwave bacon rack or a glass pie plate. In my microwave, 5 minutes on High (1 minute per slice) is about right, but microwave power varies.

Preheat your electric tabletop grill.

Put the onion, cranberries, garlic, pepper, and celery in your food processor with the S-blade in place, and pulse to chop everything to a medium consistency. Add the ground beef, oat bran, egg, Splenda, and gingerroot, and pulse again to combine. Form the mixture—it will be pretty soft—into 5 burgers. Put them on the grill, and set a timer for 6 minutes.

While the burgers are cooking, go check the bacon. If it's still a little flabby, give it another minute or so; it should be crisp. Drain the bacon if needed, and break each strip into 2 or 3 pieces to fit on top of the burgers.

When the 6 minutes are up, open your grill but do not remove the burgers. Arrange the bacon on the burgers and top each burger with cheddar cheese. Now, using a coffee mug or any other random, heat-resistant kitchen object that's handy, prop the lid of your grill up so that it's above the burgers and close to, but not touching, the cheese. Let the burgers cook for another minute or two to melt the cheese, then serve.

Yield: 5 servings, each with 8 grams of carbohydrates and 1 gram of fiber, for a total of 7 grams of usable carbs and 42 grams of protein.

Note: Cranberries are one of the very few foods that are still strictly seasonal—they're only available in the fall. However, they freeze brilliantly; just toss a plastic bag of them in the deep freeze, and it will live there happily for months. So pick up a few extra bags during the Thanksgiving shopping season and enjoy these burgers all year long.

☺ Ham and Pork Burgers

These are sort of plain and simple, but my husband loves them. This is a good recipe to help you use up leftover ham, should you have any on hand—but of course, you can also buy a chunk of precooked ham at the grocery store.

> 1/2 pound cooked ham, cut into chunks (250 g)
>
> 3/4 pound boneless pork loin, cut into chunks (750 g)
>
> 2 tablespoons oat bran
>
> 2 tablespoons heavy cream
>
> 1 egg
>
> 1/2 teaspoon pepper

Preheat your electric tabletop grill.

Plunk the ham, pork loin, oat bran, cream, egg, and pepper in a food processor with the S-blade in place, and pulse until the meat is finely ground. Form into 4 burgers, and put them in the grill. Cook for 6 to 7 minutes, and serve.

Yield: 4 servings, each with no more than 5 grams of carbohydrates (less, if you use really low-carb ham) and 1 gram of fiber, for a total of no more than 4 grams of usable carbs and 28 grams of protein.

⊕ Orange Lamb Burgers

Don't bother grinding your own lamb in your food processor; I tried this, and it came out a bit gristly. Buy ground lamb, instead. If you can't find ground lamb at your grocery store, ask the nice meat guy.

1/4 large sweet red onion

2 cloves garlic or 1 teaspoon minced garlic

1 pound ground lamb (500 g)

1 teaspoon ground cumin

1 1/2 tablespoons soy sauce

2 teaspoons grated orange zest

2 tablespoons orange juice

2 tablespoons chopped cilantro

1/4 teaspoon salt

1/2 teaspoon pepper

Preheat your electric tabletop grill.

Either chop the red onion and the garlic to a medium-fine consistency in your food processor, using the S-blade, or cut 'em up with a knife. Then put them and the lamb, cumin, soy sauce, orange zest, orange juice, cilantro, salt, and pepper in a big bowl. Using clean hands, smoosh everything together until it's all very well blended. Form the mixture into 4 burgers, and put them on the grill. Cook for 7 minutes, and serve.

Yield: 4 servings, each with 3 grams of carbohydrates, a trace of fiber, and 20 grams of protein.

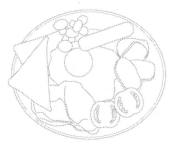

☉ Thai Burgers

Boy are these good! If you can't find fish sauce, you can substitute soy sauce and this will still taste fine.

   1 1/2 pounds boneless pork loin, cut into chunks (750 g)

   1 1/2 teaspoons lemon juice

   1 tablespoon chili garlic paste

   1 clove garlic or 1/2 teaspoon minced garlic

   4 scallions, with the roots and the tops cut off

      (leave the crisp part of the green!)

   4-ounce can mushrooms, drained (125 g)

   1 tablespoon fish sauce

   2 tablespoons fresh cilantro

   3 tablespoons lime juice

   1/2 cup mayonnaise (100 ml)

Preheat your electric tabletop grill.

Put the pork loin, lemon juice, garlic paste, garlic, scallions, mushrooms, fish sauce, and cilantro in a food processor with the S-blade in place. Pulse until the meat is finely ground and everything is well-combined. Form the mixture into 6 burgers, and put them on the grill. Cook for 6 to 7 minutes.

While the burgers are cooking, stir the lime juice (bottled works fine) into the mayonnaise. When the burgers are done, top each one with a dollop of the lime mayonnaise, and serve.

Yield: 6 servings, each with 4 grams of carbohydrates and 1 gram of fiber, for a total of 3 grams of usable carbs and 24 grams of protein.

Luau Burgers

Again, all those ingredients make this look intimidating, but it's really just a matter of assembling everything in the food processor and chopping it together.

1 pound boneless pork loin (500 g)
1/4 medium onion, cut into chunks
1/2 green pepper, cut into chunks
1 1/2 teaspoons grated gingerroot
1/2 teaspoon minced garlic or 1 clove garlic, crushed
1 tablespoon soy sauce
1 egg
1/4 cup crushed pork rinds, plain or barbeque flavor (30 g)
1/2 teaspoon pepper
1/2 teaspoon salt
1/4 cup canned crushed pineapple in unsweetened juice (50 g)
1 tablespoon tomato sauce
1/2 teaspoon blackstrap molasses
1/2 teaspoon Splenda
1/2 teaspoon spicy brown mustard

Preheat your electric tabletop grill.

Place the pork, onion, pepper, gingerroot, garlic, soy sauce, egg, pork rinds, pepper, and salt in a food processor with the S-blade in place. (You'll need a full-size food processor; this overwhelmed my little one!) Pulse until the meat is finely ground. Add the pineapple and pulse to mix.

Form into 5 burgers—the mixture will be quite soft —and slap 'em on the grill. Set a timer for 6 minutes.

While the burgers are cooking, mix together the tomato sauce, molasses, Splenda, and mustard. When the 6 minutes are up, open the grill, spread the tomato sauce mixture evenly over the burgers, then close the grill and cook for 1 more minute. Serve.

Yield: 5 servings, each with 5 grams of carbohydrates and 1 gram of fiber, for a total of 4 grams of usable carbs and 22 grams of protein.

✯ These are low calorie, too! Just 178 calories per serving.

◔ Chili Burgers

All the long-simmered flavor of chili in a fast-and-easy burger.

1 pound ground beef (500 g)

1 cup canned tomatoes with green chilies (225 ml)

1/2 medium onion, finely minced

2 cloves garlic, crushed

1 tablespoon chili powder

2 tablespoons crushed barbecue-flavor pork rinds

1 tablespoon tomato paste

1 tablespoon salt or Vege-Sal

4 ounces cheddar cheese, sliced (120 g)

Sour cream (optional)

Preheat your electric tabletop grill.

Plunk the beef, tomatoes, onion, garlic, chili powder, pork rinds, tomato paste, and salt into a bowl, and using clean hands, smoosh it all together until everything is thoroughly combined. Form this mixture into 4 patties, put them on the grill, and cook for 5 minutes.

When the 5 minutes are up, open your grill but do not remove the burgers. Top each with a slice of cheddar cheese and use whatever heat-proof kitchen object you have on hand to prop the lid of the grill open slightly for a minute or so. Let the cheese melt and serve with a dollop of sour cream, if you like.

Yield: 4 servings, each with 6 grams of carbohydrates and 1 gram of fiber, for a total of 5 grams of usable carbs and 28 grams of protein. Add 1 gram of carbs and 1 gram of protein if you use the sour cream.

Variation: These would be great with a big, simple green salad with cucumbers, green peppers, and a few tomato slices, tossed with ranch dressing.

◷ Crunchy Peking Burgers

1/2 cup canned water chestnuts, drained (80 g)

2 scallions

1 pound ground beef (500 g)

1/4 cup soy sauce (50 ml)

2 tablespoons dry sherry

1 teaspoon Splenda

1 teaspoon minced garlic or 2 cloves garlic, crushed

1/2 teaspoon grated gingerroot

Sauce

1 1/2 tablespoons low-sugar apricot preserves

1 teaspoon soy sauce

1/4 teaspoon grated gingerroot

Preheat your electric tabletop grill.

Chop the water chestnuts a bit, and slice the scallions. Put them in a mixing bowl with all the other burger ingredients, and, using clean hands, mix them well. Form into 4 burgers, and put them on the grill. Cook for 5 minutes.

While the burgers are cooking, mix together the preserves, soy sauce, and gingerroot in a small dish. When the burgers are done, top each with a teaspoon of sauce, and serve.

Yield: 4 servings, each with 7 grams of carbohydrates and 1 gram of fiber, for a total of 6 grams of usable carbs and 20 grams of protein.

⊕ Many-Pepper Burgers

Burger recipes don't get much simpler than this one!

> 1 pound ground beef (500 g)
>
> 2 1/2 tablespoons Many-Pepper Steak Seasoning (see page 218)

Preheat your electric tabletop grill.

In a mixing bowl, use clean hands to mix the ground beef and seasoning together. Form into 3 or 4 burgers, and cook them on the grill for 5 to 6 minutes.

Yield: 3 or 4 servings. Assuming 3 servings, each will have 1 gram of carbohydrates, a trace of fiber, and 25 grams of protein.

⊕ All-American Turkey Burgers

How spicy these are will depend on what sort of hot sauce you use. They're really good with coleslaw (see the recipe for Coleslaw Dressing on page 217).

> 1 pound ground turkey (500 g)
>
> 1/2 medium onion, finely chopped
>
> 1 stalk celery, finely chopped
>
> 1 teaspoon dried thyme
>
> 1 tablespoon low-carbohydrate barbecue sauce, homemade
>   or purchased
>
> 1 teaspoon hot sauce
>
> 2 teaspoons Worcestershire sauce

Preheat your electric tabletop grill.

Simply combine everything, and form the mixture into 3 burgers. Throw 'em on the grill, cook for 5 minutes, and serve.

Yield: 3 servings. The carb count will vary a bit depending on what barbecue sauce you use, but should be in the neighborhood of 4 grams of carbohydrates and 1 gram of fiber, for a total of 3 grams of usable carbs and 27 grams of protein.

chapter four

15~Minute Poultry

You'll find that most of these recipes depend upon the ubiquitous boneless, skinless chicken breast. There's a reason for this: It's nearly impossible to cook chicken on the bone in 15 minutes or less! And even with boneless, skinless chicken breasts, it's helpful, in a fair number of recipes, to pound them a little to make them thinner and an even thickness all over. This is very easy to do and takes no more than 15 to 30 seconds per breast—time well spent if it cuts 5 minutes off the cooking time. Once you've beaten a chicken breast flat a few times, you'll wonder why you've never done it before.

☺ Lemon Chicken

This Vietnamese-influenced dish has a subtle lemon-garlic flavor that combines beautifully with the spicy tart-sweet dipping sauce. And even including making the dipping sauce, this is done within our 15-minute time limit!

> 1 1/2 pounds boneless, skinless chicken breast (750 g)
>
> 1 tablespoon plus 1 teaspoon lemon juice
>
> 2 teaspoons garlic
>
> 1 tablespoon plus 1 teaspoon Splenda
>
> 2 teaspoons fish sauce (nuoc mam)
>
> 1/2 teaspoon pepper
>
> Oil
>
> Nuoc Cham dipping sauce (see page 214)

First, put the chicken breasts, one at a time, in a heavy zipper-lock bag, and use any blunt object available to beat them until they're 1/2 inch (1 cm) thick all over. Put them on a plate after they're beaten into submission.

Mix together the lemon juice, garlic, Splenda, fish sauce, and pepper, and pour the mixture evenly over the chicken breasts, turning them to make sure all sides get coated. Heat a tablespoon or two of oil in a heavy skillet over medium-high heat, and add the chicken breasts. Sauté for 4 to 5 minutes per side, or until cooked through.

While the chicken is sautéing, throw together the Nuoc Cham—this takes maybe two minutes!

In the last minute or so, pour the lemon juice mixture remaining on the plate into the skillet, turning the breasts to once again make sure both sides are coated. Heat for 1 minute and remove to serving plates. Serve with a little pool or dish of Nuoc Cham to dip bites of chicken in.

Yield: 4 servings, each with 6 grams of carbohydrate, a trace of fiber, and 38 grams of protein.

☺ Singing Chicken

This is another Vietnamese dish, and it is definitely for those who enjoy breathing fire. I'm a big fan of hot food, and this dish had me sweating by halfway through the meal. Delicious! Broccoli goes nicely with this.

2 to 3 tablespoons vegetable oil, preferably peanut

1 tablespoon grated gingerroot

1 teaspoon minced garlic or 2 cloves garlic, crushed

1 1/2 pounds boneless, skinless chicken breast,
    cut crosswise into thin slices* (750 g)

2 tablespoons Splenda

1/4 cup soy sauce (50 ml)

1 teaspoon fish sauce (nuoc mam)

3/4 cup dry white wine (170 ml)

1 fresh jalapeño, or 2 or 3 little red chilies, finely minced

1 teaspoon pepper

Guar or xanthan

* This is easiest if the meat is half-frozen.

Have the chicken sliced, the ingredients measured, the pepper minced, and everything standing by and ready to go before starting to cook—once you start stir-frying, this goes very quickly.

Put a wok or heavy skillet over high heat. Add the oil, let it heat for a minute or so, then add the ginger and garlic. Stir for 1 minute to flavor the oil. Add the chicken, and stir-fry for 1 to 2 minutes. Add the Splenda, soy sauce, fish sauce, white wine, jalapeño, and pepper, stirring often, for 7 to 8 minutes or until the chicken is cooked through. Thicken pan juices very slightly with guar or xanthan, and serve.

Yield: 3 or 4 servings. Assuming 4 servings, each will have 4 grams of carbohydrates, a trace of fiber, and 39 grams of protein.

◷ Crispy Skillet BBQ Chicken

Add some slaw made from bagged coleslaw mix, and supper is served.

> 1 1/2 pounds boneless, skinless chicken breast (750 g)
>
> Sprinkle-on barbecue dry rub or "soul" seasoning
>
> 1/2 cup crushed barbecue-flavor pork rinds (70 g)
>
> 2 tablespoons oil (30 ml)

One at a time, pound the chicken breasts until they're about 1/2 inch (1 cm) thick all over. If necessary, cut the breasts into 4 servings. Sprinkle both sides of each piece liberally with the seasoning. Then sprinkle each side of each serving with 1 tablespoon of the pork rind crumbs, and press them onto the surface with a clean palm.

Heat the oil in a large, heavy-bottomed skillet over medium-high heat. Add the chicken breasts and sauté for 5 to 6 minutes per side, or until crispy and cooked through. Serve. This is great with any sort of salad or coleslaw as a side.

Yield: 4 servings. This has no carbs to speak of (maybe a tiny trace from the seasoning), no fiber, and 44 grams of protein per serving.

◷ Aegean Chicken

The minute I told my sister about this, she started hounding me for the recipe.

> 1 1/2 pounds boneless, skinless chicken breast (750 g)
>
> 1/4 cup olive oil (50 ml)
>
> 4 ounces kasseri cheese, sliced (120 g)
>
> 8 tablespoons tapenade
>
> 1/4 cup dry white wine (50 ml)
>
> 2 cloves garlic

One at a time, pound the chicken breasts till they're 1/4 inch (5 mm) thick all over. Cut the breasts into 6 servings, if necessary. Sauté them in the olive oil over medium-high heat. When they're turning golden on the bottom, turn them, and lay the slices of kasseri over them. Let them cook another 2 to 3 minutes, or until the cheese is starting to melt. Spread the tapenade over the breasts, and add the wine to the skillet. Let the whole thing cook for another minute or two, just to warm the tapenade and make sure the chicken is cooked through. Remove the chicken to serving plates, add the garlic to the wine left in the skillet, stir the whole thing and let it boil for a minute or so, and pour it over the chicken before serving.

Yield: 6 servings, each with just 2 grams of carbohydrates, a trace of fiber, and 40 grams of protein.

☺ Cashew Crusted Chicken

Since cashews are a relatively high-carb nut, this is just a light coating—but very flavorful. You can find raw cashews at most health food stores.

> 2/3 cup raw cashew pieces (70 g)
>
> 1/4 teaspoon salt
>
> 1/2 teaspoon pepper
>
> 1/4 teaspoon paprika
>
> 1 1/2 pounds boneless, skinless chicken breast (750 g)
>
> 1 egg
>
> 2 to 3 tablespoons butter

First, put the cashew pieces in a food processor with the S-blade in place, and grind them to a fine texture. Dump them out onto a plate and add the salt, pepper, and paprika, mixing the whole thing well. Set aside.

Pound the chicken breasts until they're 1/2 inch (1 cm) thick all over. Cut into 4 servings if necessary.

Break the egg into another plate with a rim around it. (A pie plate would work well.) Now, dip each chicken breast piece into the egg, then into the cashew mixture, coating both sides.

Melt the butter in a heavy skillet over medium to medium-high heat, and add the chicken. Sauté until it's golden on both sides and cooked through, about 5 minutes per side.

Yield: 4 servings, each with 6 grams of carbohydrates and 1 gram of fiber, for a total of 5 grams of usable carbs and 33 grams of protein.

⊕ Chicken Breast Italiano

Ridiculously easy, especially considering how good it tastes! This is great with one of the cauliflower "risottos" as a side dish (see page 175).

>   1 1/2 pounds boneless, skinless chicken breast (750 g)
>
>   2 tablespoons olive oil
>
>   1/3 cup bottled Italian salad dressing (70 ml)

In a heavy-bottomed skillet, sauté the chicken breasts in the olive oil over medium heat. Cover them while they're cooking, and turn them after 6 to 7 minutes. When both sides are golden and the chicken is cooked most of the way through, add the Italian dressing, turn the breasts to coat both sides, and let the whole thing cook for another 2 to 3 minutes before serving.

Yield: 4 servings, each with 2 grams of carbohydrates, no fiber, and 38 grams of protein.

⊕ Chicken Tenders

Good for when you're having fast-food cravings or the kids are nagging for "normal" food. You really can make these in 15 minutes—because the pieces are small, they cook very quickly.

>   1 pound boneless, skinless chicken breast (500 g)
>
>   1 egg
>
>   1 tablespoon water
>
>   3/4 cup low-carb bake mix (100 g)
>
>   1/2 teaspoon salt
>
>   1/4 teaspoon pepper
>
>   1/3 cup oil (70 ml)

Cut the chicken breasts into pieces about 1 inch wide and 2 inches long. Beat the egg with the water in a bowl. On a plate, combine the bake mix with the salt and pepper. Heat the oil in a heavy skillet over medium-high heat.

Dip each chicken piece in the egg wash, then roll it in the seasoned bake mix, and drop it in the hot oil. Fry these until golden all over, and serve with one of the dipping sauces in the Condiments, Sauces, Dressings, and Seasonings chapter (see page 211).

Yield: 4 servings, each with 5 grams of carbohydrates and 2 grams of fiber, for a total of 3 grams of usable carbs (exclusive of the dipping sauces) and 40 grams of protein.

☉ Seriously Spicy Citrus Chicken

You could cut back on the red pepper flakes if you'd like to make Moderately Spicy Citrus Chicken.

> 1 1/2 pounds boneless, skinless chicken breast (750 g)
>
> 1/4 cup olive oil (50 ml)
>
> 1/2 cup lime juice (100 ml)
>
> 1/4 cup lemon juice (50 ml)
>
> 1 tablespoon plus 1 teaspoon red pepper flakes
>
> 1 tablespoon plus 1 teaspoon minced garlic
>
> 1 tablespoon plus 1 teaspoon grated gingerroot
>
> 1/4 cup Splenda (30 g)
>
> 4 scallions, finely sliced
>
> 2 tablespoons chopped cilantro

Cut the chicken into 4 servings, if necessary. Sauté the chicken in the olive oil over medium-high heat, with a tilted lid. While it's sautéing, mix together the lime juice, lemon juice, red pepper flakes, garlic, gingerroot, and Splenda. After the chicken has turned golden on both sides (about 4 to 5 minutes per side), pour the lime juice mixture into the skillet and turn the breasts over to coat both sides. Sauté for another 2 to 3 minutes on each side, then move the chicken to serving plates, scraping the liquid from the pan over the chicken. Scatter sliced scallions and chopped cilantro over each portion, and serve.

Yield: 4 servings, each with 8 grams of carbohydrates and 1 gram of fiber, for a total of 7 grams of usable carbs and 32 grams of protein.

☉ Apricot-Bourbon Chicken

This is amazing—as good as anything I've ever had in a fancy restaurant—yet it's fast enough to make on a weeknight after work! I like the Saffron "Rice" (see page 177) as a side with this.

 2 pounds boneless, skinless chicken breasts (1 kg)

 3 tablespoons butter

 1/2 cup chopped pecans (50 g)

 1/4 cup low-sugar apricot preserves (50 ml)

 1/4 cup bourbon (50 ml)

 2 tablespoons plain tomato sauce

 2 teaspoons spicy brown or Dijon mustard

 1/2 teaspoon minced garlic or 1 clove garlic, crushed

 1/4 cup minced onion (30 g)

 3 scallions, thinly sliced

First, pound the chicken breasts until they're 1/2 inch (1 cm) thick all over, and cut into 6 portions. Brown them in 2 tablespoons of butter in a large, heavy skillet over high heat.

While the breasts are browning, melt the last tablespoon of butter in a small, heavy skillet, and stir in the pecans. Stir them over medium-high heat for a few minutes, until they begin to turn golden. Turn off the heat (and if yours is an electric stove, remove from the burner to prevent scorching) and reserve.

Stir together the preserves, bourbon, tomato sauce, mustard, garlic, and onion. When the chicken is light golden on both sides, pour this mixture into the skillet. Turn the chicken over once or twice, to coat both sides with the sauce. Cover with a tilted lid, and let it simmer for about 5 minutes, or until cooked through.

Serve with the sauce spooned over each portion, and top each with the toasted pecans and sliced scallions.

Yield: 6 servings, each with 7 grams of carbohydrates and 1 gram of fiber, for a total of 6 grams of usable carbs and 35 grams of protein.

☐ Chicken Breasts L'Orange

Chicken combines so well with all sorts of fruit flavors, and this dish is sure to be a hit with the whole family.

1 ¹/₂ pounds boneless, skinless chicken breast (750 g)

¹/₄ cup oil (50 ml)

¹/₃ cup orange juice (75 ml)

2 tablespoons Splenda

2 teaspoons cider vinegar

¹/₄ teaspoon blackstrap molasses

1 teaspoon spicy brown or Dijon mustard

1 teaspoon minced garlic or 2 cloves garlic, crushed

Salt and pepper

Cut the chicken breasts into 4 portions, and brown them in the oil in a large, heavy skillet over high heat. While that's happening, mix together the orange juice, Splenda, vinegar, molasses, mustard, and garlic.

When the chicken is light golden on both sides, add the orange juice mixture to the skillet. Simmer the chicken for another 7 to 8 minutes, turning once. Salt and pepper to taste, and serve.

Yield: 4 servings, each with 4 grams of carbohydrates, a trace of fiber, and 38 grams of protein.

☉ Chicken with Asparagus and Gruyère

> 1 1/2 pounds boneless, skinless chicken breast (750 g)
>
> 1 tablespoon butter
>
> 1 pound asparagus (500 g)
>
> 1 tablespoon dry white wine
>
> 1 tablespoon lemon juice
>
> Salt and pepper
>
> 4 ounces gruyère, thinly sliced (120 g)

First, pound the chicken breasts until they're 1/4 inch (5 mm) thick all over. Cut into 4 portions.

Melt the butter in a large, heavy skillet over medium-high heat, and start browning the chicken.

While that's happening, snap the ends off the asparagus where they break naturally. Put the asparagus in a microwaveable casserole or lay it in a glass pie plate. Add a couple of tablespoons of water, and cover. (Use plastic wrap or a plate to cover if you're using a pie plate.) Microwave on High for 3 to 4 minutes.

When the chicken is golden on both sides, add the wine and the lemon juice to the skillet and turn the chicken breasts to coat both sides. Salt and pepper lightly. Turn the burner to medium-low heat and let the chicken continue to cook until the asparagus is done microwaving.

Remove the asparagus from the microwave and drain. Lay the asparagus spears over the chicken, dividing equally between the portions. Cover each with gruyère, and cover the skillet with a tilted lid. Continue cooking a few minutes, just until the cheese is melted. Serve.

Yield: 4 servings, each with 3 grams of carbohydrates and 1 gram of fiber, for a total of 2 grams of usable carbs and 38 grams of protein.

⊕ Parmesan Chicken Breasts

Those of you who bought my first cookbook, *500 Low-Carb Recipes*, will recognize this recipe as being quite similar to Heroin Wings. However, Heroin Wings take well over an hour, and this is quite quick.

1 1/2 pounds boneless, skinless chicken breast (750 g)

1 cup grated Parmesan cheese* (150 g)

4 teaspoons dried oregano

1 teaspoon garlic powder

1 teaspoon paprika

1 teaspoon pepper

2 eggs

4 tablespoons butter

* Use the cheap stuff in the round, green shaker for this.

Pound the chicken breasts till they're 1/4 inch (5 mm) thick, and cut into 6 portions. Set aside.

Combine the cheese with the oregano, garlic, paprika, and pepper on a plate. On another plate or in a shallow bowl, beat the eggs. Dip the chicken in the egg and then the cheese mixture, coating both sides well.

Melt the butter in a heavy skillet over medium-low heat (higher heat will scorch the cheese), and sauté for 4 to 5 minutes per side, or until cooked through.

Yield: 6 servings, each with 2 grams of carbohydrates and 1 gram of fiber, for a total of 1 gram of usable carbs and 33 grams of protein.

☺ The Only 15-Minute Wings I Could Figure Out

Because I love chicken wings and know that lots of other folks do, too, I tried several ways of cooking them, trying to come up with a way to cook a halfway decent wing within our 15-minute time frame. I'm here to tell you it ain't easy. Frying them took too long and left a big mess. Baked wings were done within 15 minutes if I cranked my oven all the way to 500°F (240°C, Gas Mark 9)—but preheating the oven that hot added extra 15 minutes to the process.

Finally I hit on cooking them in my electric tabletop grill, and it worked! My wings were done through, and while they weren't as wonderfully crunchy as oven-baked wings, they were acceptably crisp.

> Chicken wings—as many as will fit in your grill
> (mine fits about 8 whole wings)
> Sprinkle-on seasoning of your choice (dry rub barbecue
> seasoning, jerk seasoning, lemon pepper,
> Cajun seasoning, Creole seasoning
> —or just salt and pepper, if you prefer)

Plug your grill in. Do not wait for it to heat up—you need every second of cooking time you can get. Arrange the wings on the grill, pulling them open (extending them at the joints) so they lay as flat as possible on the grill. (Obviously, if you're using cut-up wing "drummettes" this won't be necessary.) Fit as many on the grill as you can. Then sprinkle them with your chosen seasoning, and close the grill. Press down gently on the top of the grill, to make sure that the grill is in firm contact with as much of the surface of the wings as possible. Cook for 13 to 15 minutes, and serve.

Yield: How many servings you get will depend on the size of your grill. Each wing will have a negligible amount of carbs, no fiber, and 9 grams of protein. (That's for whole wings; figure roughly half that for each "drummette.")

☉ Lemon-Glazed Turkey Cutlets

Turkey cutlets—slices of turkey breast less than 1/4 inch (5 mm) thick—are good for cooks in a hurry because they take almost no time to cook through. They're pretty bland by themselves, however, and can easily turn dry and tough. But they take beautifully to this tart-sweet lemon glaze.

3 turkey cutlets, about 4 ounces (120 g) each

1 tablespoon olive oil

1 tablespoon lemon juice

1 tablespoon dry sherry

2 teaspoons Splenda

1/2 teaspoon soy sauce

Guar or xanthan

3 scallions, finely sliced

In a large, heavy skillet over medium heat, brown the cutlets in the oil. While that's happening, mix together the lemon juice, sherry, Splenda, soy sauce, and just a sprinkle of guar or xanthan to thicken the mixture. When the cutlets have just a touch of golden color on each side, pour the lemon juice mixture into the skillet, and turn the cutlets over once to coat both sides. Turn the burner to medium-low, cover, and let the cutlets simmer for just a few more minutes, until the sauce reduces a little.

Serve with any glaze left in the pan scraped over the cutlets and a sliced scallion scattered over each.

Yield: 2 or 3 servings. Assuming 2 servings, each will have 4 grams of carbohydrates and 1 gram of fiber, for a total of 3 grams of usable carbs and 37 grams of protein.

☉ Mustard-Pecan Turkey Cutlets

Of all the things I've tried with turkey cutlets, this is my husband's favorite. The mustard-mayo coating keeps these from getting dry.

> 1/2 cup shelled pecans (50 g)
>
> 1 tablespoon spicy brown or Dijon mustard
>
> 3 tablespoons mayonnaise
>
> 3 turkey breast cutlets, about 4 ounces (120 g) each
>
> 1 1/2 tablespoons butter

Place the pecans in your food processor with the S-blade in place, and pulse until they're ground medium-fine. (Alternately, you could buy the pecans already ground.)

Mix together the mustard and mayonnaise, blending well.

Lay the turkey cutlets on a plate, and spread half of the mustard and mayonnaise mixture on one side. Sprinkle half of the ground pecans over the mustard and mayonnaise, and press lightly with the back of a spoon to help them stick.

Spray a large, heavy skillet with nonstick cooking spray. Place over medium-high heat. Melt the butter and add the cutlets, pecan side down. Sauté for about 4 minutes. With the cutlets still in the pan, spread the remaining mustard-mayo mixture on the uncoated sides, and sprinkle the rest of the pecans over that, once again pressing them in a bit with the back of a spoon. Flip the cutlets carefully, doing your best not to dislodge the crust. Sauté for another 5 minutes, and serve. Scrape any yummy toasted pecans that are stuck to the skillet over the cutlets before serving.

Yield: 2 or 3 servings. Assuming 2 servings, each will have 4 grams of carbohydrates and 2 grams of fiber, for a total of 2 grams of usable carbs and 39 grams of protein.

☉ Lettuce Wraps

These are currently a hot appetizer at Asian restaurants, and they're delicious—but the restaurant version usually contains an unacceptable amount of sugar. Serve these as an appetizer if you like, but I like them as a light supper. Even if you have to make the Asian Dipping Sauce, too, this comes in under the 15-minute time limit.

8-ounce can water chestnuts, drained (250 g)

1 cup sliced mushrooms (80 ml)

5 scallions, roots and limp shoot removed, cut into 2 or 3 pieces each

3 tablespoons soy sauce

2 tablespoons Splenda

1/2 teaspoon blackstrap molasses

1 1/2 teaspoons minced garlic or 3 cloves of garlic, crushed

1 1/2 teaspoons rice vinegar

3 tablespoons oil

1 pound ground chicken (500 g)

Guar or xanthan

Iceberg or leaf lettuce

Asian Dipping Sauce (see page 213)

Place the water chestnuts, mushrooms, and scallions in your food processor with the S-blade in place. Pulse just enough to chop everything to a medium consistency.

Combine the soy sauce, Splenda, blackstrap molasses, garlic, and rice vinegar. Set aside.

Heat the oil in a wok or large skillet over highest heat. Add the chicken and stir-fry, breaking it up as it cooks. When about half of the pink is gone from the chicken, add the chopped vegetables and stir-fry everything together for a few more minutes. When the chicken is cooked through, stir in the seasoning mixture and let everything cook together for just another minute or so. Thicken the pan juices just a little with guar or xanthan, and serve.

To eat this, you wrap spoonfuls of the meat mixture in lettuce leaves, dip the rolls in the Asian Dipping Sauce, then eat them by hand. The tidiest way to do this is to take a whole, firm head of iceberg lettuce, and slice a good 2-inch-thick (5 cm thick) slab off the side, making "lettuce cups"—you can do this all over the head, leaving the inside of the head for salad. However, there's no reason not to use leaf lettuce if you prefer it.

Yield: Figure this is 6 servings as an appetizer, each with 10 grams of carbohydrates and 2 grams of fiber, for a total of 8 grams of usable carbs (exclusive of the dipping sauce) and 25 grams of protein, which is a pretty filling appetizer!

Figure this is 4 servings as a main course, each with 15 grams of carbohydrates and 3 grams of fiber, for a total of 12 grams of usable carbs (again, exclusive of the dipping sauce) and 37 grams of protein.

☉ Easy Mexicali Chicken

How simple this is! Yet you know the whole family will like it. Just remember to read the labels to get the lowest-carb salsa.

> 1 1/2 pounds boneless, skinless chicken breast (750 g)
> 2 tablespoons oil
> 4 ounces Monterey Jack, pepper Jack, or shredded Mexican cheese blend, as you prefer (120 g)
> 1/2 cup mild, medium, or hot salsa, as you prefer (100 ml)

Pound the chicken breasts to 1/2 inch (1 cm) thick, and divide into portions, if needed.

Place your large, heavy skillet over medium-high heat, add the oil, and sauté the chicken breasts for about 5 minutes, or until the bottom is golden. Turn, and sauté for another 3 to 4 minutes. Top the chicken with the cheese, turn the heat down to medium-low, cover the skillet, and let the whole thing cook for another 3 to 4 minutes, or until the cheese is melted.

While the cheese is melting, put the salsa in a microwaveable dish and nuke it for a minute at 50 percent power.

Remove the chicken to serving plates, top with the salsa, and serve. You could add a dollop of sour cream if you like, or maybe some chopped fresh cilantro, but it's not really necessary.

Yield: 4 or 5 servings. Assuming 4 servings, each will have 2 grams of carbohydrates and 1 gram of fiber, for a total of 1 gram of usable carbs and 45 grams of protein.

☉ Chicken Liver Sauté

The worst possible thing you can do to liver of any kind is overcook it, which makes chicken livers an ideal candidate for a super-fast gourmet supper. The cauliflower rice is optional with this, but it takes very little extra time, adds only 1 gram of extra carbs to a serving, and makes this seem more like a meal.

> 1/2 head cauliflower (optional)
>
> 8 ounces chicken livers (250 g)
>
> 4 ounces sliced mushrooms (120 g)
>
> 1/4 medium onion
>
> 1 tablespoon butter
>
> 1/2 teaspoon minced garlic or 1 clove garlic, crushed
>
> 1/2 teaspoon ground rosemary*
>
> 1/4 cup dry sherry (50 ml)
>
> 1/2 teaspoon lemon juice
>
> Salt and pepper
>
> Guar or xanthan

* You can use a teaspoon of dried rosemary needles instead, and it will taste good, but you'll have little tough needles in your food.

If you want cauliflower rice to serve the chicken livers on, make that first. Run the cauliflower through the shredding blade of your food processor, put it in a microwaveable casserole with a lid, add a couple of tablespoons of water, cover it, and microwave it on High for 7 minutes. If the cauliflower is done cooking before you're quite done with your livers, *remove the lid*. This will let the steam out and stop the cooking. Otherwise you'll get a white mush that bears little resemblance to rice, or even cauliflower.

Okay, you're ready to deal with the livers. Cut each liver into 3 or 4 chunks. We're assuming you bought presliced mushrooms, but if you didn't, slice them now. Take the onion quarter, cut it in half again (making two eighths), and then slice it as thin as you can.

Melt the butter in a large, heavy skillet over medium-high heat. Add the livers, mushrooms, onions, and garlic, and stir-fry until the mushrooms are starting to change color and most of the pink is gone from the livers. Add the rosemary, sherry, lemon juice, and a little salt and pepper, and let it all simmer for just 1 to 2 minutes. Thicken the pan liquid slightly with guar or xanthan, and serve, with or without cauliflower rice.

Yield: 2 servings. Without the cauliflower rice, each serving will have 8 grams of carbohydrates and 1 gram of fiber, for a total of 7 grams of usable carbs and 22 grams of protein.

If you serve it with the cauliflower rice, each serving will have 10 grams of carbohydrates and 2 grams of fiber, for a total of 8 grams of usable carbs and 22 grams of protein.

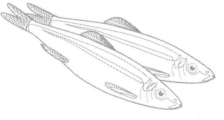

chapter five

15~Minute Fish and Seafood

If you're trying to eat low-carb and to be as healthy as possible on a tight schedule, you just can't do any better than fish. Of course we know fish is wonderful for us, but it's also to our advantage that it's hard to find a fish recipe that calls for more than 15 minutes' cooking time!

Indeed, the only thing I can think of to say against fish is that it is often expensive. Around here, the fish we eat most often are catfish, tilapia, and whiting, for the simple reason that they're the fish that are cheapest, at least here in the Midwest.

However, fish are frequently interchangeable in recipes, so if you prefer sole, orange roughy, cod, flounder, or what-have-you, don't hesitate to try them. There's no reason why they shouldn't work out fine, with a little adjustment of time for thicker or thinner fillets.

◷ Shrimp Stewed in Curry Butter

Don't bother with napkins, just put the roll of paper towels on the table
—this is messy! It's delicious, though.

> 6 tablespoons butter
>
> 2 teaspoons curry powder
>
> 1 teaspoon minced garlic or 2 cloves garlic, crushed
>
> 24 large, raw, "easy peel" shrimp

Melt the butter in a large, heavy skillet over lowest heat. Stir in the curry powder
and garlic, then add the shrimp in a single layer. Cook for 3 to 5 minutes per side, or
until the shrimp are pink right through. Transfer to serving plates, and scrape the
extra curry butter over them.

Yield: 2 servings, each with 2 grams of carbohydrates, 1 gram of fiber (if you lick
up every last drop of the curry-garlic butter), for a total of a bit less than 1 gram
of usable carbs per serving and 15 grams of protein.

◷ Saigon Shrimp

Vietnamese style—hot and a little sweet.

> Scant 1/2 teaspoon salt
>
> Scant 1/2 teaspoon pepper
>
> 1 1/2 teaspoons Splenda
>
> 3 scallions
>
> 4 tablespoons peanut or canola oil
>
> 1 pound large shrimp, shelled and deveined (500 g)
>
> 1 1/2 teaspoons chili garlic paste
>
> 2 teaspoons minced garlic

Mix together the salt, pepper, and Splenda in a small dish or cup. Slice the
scallions thinly, and set them aside. Gather all the ingredients except the scallions
together—the actual cooking of this dish is lightning fast!

In a wok or heavy skillet over highest heat, heat the oil. Add the shrimp, and stir-fry for 2 to 3 minutes, or until they're about two-thirds pink. Add the chili garlic paste and garlic, and keep stir-frying. When the shrimp are pink all over and all the way through, sprinkle the salt, pepper, and Splenda mixture over them, and stir for just another 10 seconds or so. Turn off the heat and divide the shrimp between 3 serving plates. Top each serving with a scattering of sliced scallion, and serve.

Yield: 3 servings, each with 2 grams of carbohydrates and 1 gram of fiber, for a total of 1 gram of usable carbs and 25 grams of protein.

✳ This dish comes in at a low 288 calories a serving.

🕑 Shrimp in Brandy Cream

Wow—sheer elegance. And done in a flash!

> 1 pound shrimp, shelled and deveined (500 g)
> 4 tablespoons butter
> 1/3 cup brandy (70 ml)
> 3/4 cup heavy cream (170 ml)
> Guar or xanthan (optional)

Sauté the shrimp in the butter over medium-high heat until cooked through—4 to 5 minutes. Add the brandy, turn up the heat, and let it boil hard for a minute or so, to reduce. Stir in the cream, and heat through. Thicken the sauce a bit with guar or xanthan if you like, then serve.

Yield: 3 or 4 servings. Assuming 3 servings, each will have 2 grams of carbohydrates, no fiber, and 26 grams of protein.

☺ Salmon in Ginger Cream

All the goodness of salmon in an elegant sauce.

> 2 tablespoons butter
>
> 2 pieces salmon fillet, 6 ounces (150 g) each, skin still attached
>
> 1 teaspoon minced garlic or 2 cloves garlic, crushed
>
> 2 scallions, finely minced
>
> 2 tablespoons chopped cilantro
>
> 4 tablespoons dry white wine
>
> 2 tablespoons grated gingerroot
>
> 4 tablespoons sour cream
>
> Salt and pepper

Melt the butter in a heavy skillet over medium-low heat, and start sautéing the salmon in it—you want to sauté it for about 4 minutes per side.

While the fish is sautéing, crush the garlic, mince the scallions, and chop the cilantro.

When both sides of the salmon have sautéed for 4 minutes, add the wine to the skillet, cover, and let the fish cook an additional 2 minutes or so, until done through. Remove the fish to serving plates.

Add the garlic, scallions, cilantro, and ginger to the wine and butter in the skillet, turn the burner up to medium-high, and let them cook for a minute or two. Add the sour cream, stir to blend, and salt and pepper to taste. Spoon the sauce over the fish, and serve.

Yield: 2 servings, each with 5 grams of carbohydrates and 1 gram of fiber, for a total of 4 grams of usable carbs and 36 grams of protein

✳ This dish also has lots of EPA—the good fat that makes salmon so heart-healthy!

☉ Buttered Salmon with Creole Seasonings

12 ounces salmon fillet, in two or three pieces (350 g)

1 teaspoon purchased Creole seasoning

1/4 teaspoon dried thyme

4 tablespoons butter

1 teaspoon minced garlic or 2 cloves garlic, minced

Sprinkle the skinless side of the salmon evenly with the Creole seasoning and thyme. Melt the butter in a heavy skillet over medium-low heat, and add the salmon, skin side down. Cook 4 to 5 minutes per side, turning carefully. Remove to serving plates, skin side down, and stir the garlic into the butter remaining in the pan. Cook for just a minute, then scrape all the garlic butter over the salmon, and serve.

Yield: 2 or 3 servings. Assuming 2 servings, each will have 2 grams of carbohydrates and a trace of fiber, for a total of 2 grams of usable carbs and 35 grams of protein.

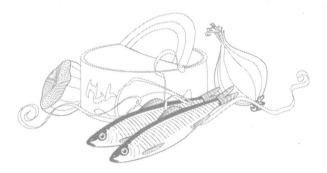

⊕ Glazed, Grilled Salmon

Of all the ways I've cooked salmon, this drew the most praise.

> 2 tablespoons Splenda
>
> 1 1/2 teaspoons dry mustard
>
> 1 tablespoon soy sauce
>
> 1 1/2 teaspoons rice vinegar
>
> 1/4 teaspoon blackstrap molasses, or the darkest molasses you can find
>
> 12 ounces salmon fillet, cut into 2 or 3 serving-size pieces (350 g)

Mix together the Splenda, mustard, soy sauce, vinegar, and molasses in a small dish. Spoon out 1 tablespoon of this mixture, and set it aside in a separate dish.

Place the salmon fillets on a plate, and pour the larger quantity of the soy sauce mixture over it, turning each fillet so that both sides come in contact with the seasonings. Let the fish sit for a few minutes—just 2 or 3—with the skinless side down in the seasonings.

Now, you get to choose how you want to cook the salmon. I do mine on a stove top grill, but you can broil it, do it in a heavy skillet sprayed with nonstick cooking spray, cook it on your electric tabletop grill, or even do it on your outdoor grill. However you cook it, it will need about 5 minutes per side (or just 5 minutes total, in an electric grill). If you choose a method that requires you to turn the salmon, turn carefully! Baste once, when turning, with the soy sauce mixture you reserved. (Don't do it after that—you want the heat to kill any raw fish germs!)

When the salmon is cooked through, remove it to serving plates and drizzle the reserved seasoning mixture over each piece before serving.

Yield: This makes 2 generous servings or 3 smaller ones. Assuming 2 servings, each will have 3 grams of carbohydrates, a trace of fiber, and 35 grams of protein.

☺ Whiting with Mexican Flavors

I made this for lunch when a friend of my husband's was visiting town, and we all agreed it was one of the best things I've ever made.

> 4 whiting fillets
>
> 2 tablespoons lime juice
>
> 3/4 teaspoon chili powder
>
> 2 tablespoons oil
>
> 1 medium onion
>
> 2 tablespoons orange juice
>
> 1/2 teaspoon Splenda
>
> 1/4 teaspoon ground cumin
>
> 1/4 teaspoon dried oregano
>
> 1 tablespoon white wine vinegar
>
> 1/2 teaspoon hot sauce
>
> Salt and pepper

Lay the whiting fillets on a plate, and sprinkle with 1 tablespoon of lime juice, turning to coat. Sprinkle the skinless sides of the fillets with chili powder.

Heat the oil in a heavy skillet over medium heat. Add the whiting fillets. Sauté for about 4 minutes per side, turning carefully, or until cooked through. Remove to a serving plate and keep warm.

Add the onions to the skillet, and turn the heat up to medium-high. Sauté the onions for a couple of minutes, until they begin to go limp. Stir in the orange juice, Splenda, cumin, oregano, vinegar, and hot sauce. Cook them all together for a minute or two. Salt and pepper to taste. Spoon the onions over the fish, and serve.

Yield: 4 servings, each with 5 grams of carbohydrates and 1 gram of fiber, for a total of 4 grams of usable carbs and 17 grams of protein.

❄ Each serving has only 162 calories!

☺ Chinese Steamed Fish

I made this with tilapia, and while it was quite tasty, it was also fragile. If you're willing to pay the difference for a firmer fish like orange roughy or cod, it will be easier to handle.

> 12 ounces fish fillets (350 g)
>
> 2 tablespoons dry sherry
>
> 1 tablespoon soy sauce
>
> 2 teaspoons grated gingerroot
>
> 1/2 teaspoon minced garlic or 1 clove garlic, crushed
>
> 1 1/2 teaspoons toasted sesame oil
>
> 1 or 2 scallions, minced (optional)

Lay the fish fillets on a piece of heavy-duty aluminum foil, and turn the edges up to form a lip.

Mix together the sherry, soy sauce, gingerroot, garlic, and sesame oil.

Fit a rack—a cake-cooling rack works nicely—into a large skillet. Pour about 1/4 inch (5 mm) of water in the bottom of the skillet, and turn the heat to high. Place the foil with the fish on it on the rack. Carefully pour the sherry mixture over the fish. Cover the pan tightly.

Cook for 5 to 7 minutes, or until the fish flakes easily. Serve with minced scallions as a garnish, if desired.

Yield: 2 servings, each with 2 grams of carbohydrates, no fiber, and 31 grams of protein.

✻ Each serving has only 195 calories!

Three Ridiculously Easy Things To Do with Catfish

(Plus One That's Only a Tiny Bit More Complicated)

You'll notice a certain similarity between these three recipes, but they all taste quite different—and quite good! Personally, I think coleslaw (with sugar-free dressing, of course) would make an ideal side dish with any of these recipes, but then again, I'm inordinately fond of coleslaw. Despite the butter, all three of these recipes come in at under 300 calories per serving, as well as being very low carb.

☺ Lemon-Pepper Catfish

> 1 pound catfish fillets (500 g)
> Lemon pepper
> 3 to 4 tablespoons butter

Sprinkle both sides of the catfish fillets liberally with lemon pepper, and let them sit for 5 minutes. Melt the butter over medium heat in a heavy skillet. Add the catfish, and sauté for about 5 minutes per side, or until cooked through, then serve.

Yield: 3 servings, each with 1 gram of carbohydrates, a trace of fiber, and 25 grams of protein.

☺ Old Bay Catfish

> 1 pound catfish fillets (500 g)
> Old Bay Seasoning*
> 3 to 4 tablespoons butter

* This is a widely available sprinkle-on seasoning; look for it in your grocery store.

Sprinkle both sides of the catfish fillets liberally with Old Bay Seasoning, and let them sit for 5 minutes. Melt the butter over medium heat in a heavy skillet. Add the catfish, and sauté for about 5 minutes per side, or until cooked through, then serve.

Yield: 3 servings, each with just a trace of carbohydrates, no fiber, and 25 grams of protein.

🕐 Creole Catfish

> 1 pound catfish fillets (500 g)
>
> Creole seasoning
>
> 3 to 4 tablespoons butter

Sprinkle both sides of the catfish fillets liberally with Creole seasoning, and let them sit for 5 minutes. Melt the butter over medium heat in a heavy skillet. Add the catfish, and sauté for about 5 minutes per side, or until cooked through, then serve.

Yield: 3 servings, each with 2 grams of carbohydrates, a trace of fiber, and 25 grams of protein.

🕐 Crunchy Creole Catfish

Nice alliteration, huh? If you have some crushed BBQ pork rinds on hand, this is a tasty elaboration on the previous catfish recipe.

> 1 pound catfish fillets (500 g)
>
> Creole seasoning
>
> 1/3 cup crushed barbeque-flavor pork rinds (50 g)
>
> 3 tablespoons butter

Sprinkle the catfish fillets liberally on both sides with Creole seasoning. Spread the pork rind crumbs on a plate, and dip both sides of each fillet in the crumbs to coat. Melt the butter in a heavy skillet over medium heat, and sauté the fillets for 4 to 5 minutes per side, or until cooked through and crispy.

Yield: 2-3 servings, each with 2 grams of carbohydrates, a trace of fiber and 46 grams of protein.

☯ Oysters en Brochette

Oysters are an oddity in the world of animal protein, in that they actually contain a few carbs of their own. Still, they're quite nutritious (loaded with zinc) and many people love them. This makes an elegant appetizer or a very light supper.

>   6 slices bacon
>
>   24 mushrooms
>
>   16 large oysters
>
>   Butter (optional)
>
>   Lemon wedges (optional)

You'll either need metal skewers for this or you'll need to think far enough ahead to put 6 bamboo skewers in water to soak for a few hours before you begin cooking.

Either way, simply skewer a slice of bacon near the end, then skewer a mushroom. Fold the strip of bacon back over, skewering it again, then add an oyster, and fold and skewer the bacon again—you're weaving the bacon in and out of the alternating mushrooms and oysters, see?

Lay the skewers on a broiler pan, and broil them close to the heat, with the broiler on Low, for about 10 minutes. Turn once or twice, until the oysters are done and the bacon's getting crisp. You can baste these with butter while they're broiling if you like, but it's not strictly necessary. Serve one skewer per customer as a first course, with lemon wedges if you like.

Yield: 3 servings, each with 8 grams of carbohydrates and 2 grams of fiber, for a total of 6 grams of usable carbs and 10 grams of protein.

Two Variations: My husband, who refers to mushrooms as "slime," likes these without the mushrooms. This cuts the carb count down to just 2 grams per serving.

If you'd like to impress the guests at your next party, you can cut strips of bacon in half and wrap each half-strip around an oyster, piercing with a toothpick to hold. Broil as above until the bacon gets crispy, and serve hot. These are called Angels on Horseback—I have no idea why—and they're a classic hot hors d'oeuvre. These will have just a trace of carbohydrates per piece.

☉ Microwaved Fish and Asparagus with Tarragon Mustard Sauce

Microwaving is a great way to cook vegetables and a great way to cook fish—so it's a natural way to cook combinations of the two.

10 asparagus spears

2 tablespoons sour cream

1 tablespoon mayonnaise

1/4 teaspoon dried tarragon

1/2 teaspoon Dijon or spicy brown mustard

12 ounces fish fillets—whiting, tilapia, sole, flounder, or any other mild white fish (350 g)

Snap the bottoms off the asparagus spears where they break naturally. Place the asparagus in a large glass pie plate, add 1 tablespoon of water, and cover by placing a plate on top. Microwave on High for 3 minutes.

While the asparagus is microwaving, stir together the sour cream, mayonnaise, tarragon, and mustard.

Remove the asparagus from the microwave, take it out of the pie plate, and set it aside. Drain the water out of the pie plate. Place the fish fillets in the pie plate, and spread 2 tablespoons of the sour cream mixture over them. Re-cover the pie plate, and microwave the fish for 3 to 4 minutes on High. Open the microwave, remove the plate from the top of the pie plate, and arrange the asparagus on top of the fish. Re-cover the pie plate, and cook for another 1 to 2 minutes on High.

Remove the pie plate from the microwave, and take the plate off. Place the fish and asparagus on serving plates. Scrape any sauce that's cooked into the pie plate over the fish and asparagus. Top each serving with the reserved sauce, and serve.

Yield: 2 servings, each with 4 grams of carbohydrates and 2 grams of fiber, for a total of 2 grams of usable carbs and 33 grams of protein.

✷ This dish also packs in 949 milligrams of potassium!

◷ California Tuna Fritters

This makes a quick and different supper out of simple canned tuna. You can make this into a few big tuna burgers, if you prefer, and cut a few minutes off the cooking time, but we really like these as little fritters.

    1 stalk celery
    6 scallions
    1/2 green pepper
    2 tablespoons chopped parsley
    1 egg
    1 tablespoon spicy brown mustard or Dijon mustard
    12 ounces canned water-pack tuna, drained (350 g)
    1/3 cup rice protein powder (30 g)
    4 to 5 tablespoons butter

Plunk the celery, scallions, pepper, parsley, egg, and mustard in a food processor with the S-blade in place, and pulse until the vegetables are chopped to a medium-fine consistency. Add the tuna and rice protein, and pulse to mix.

Spray a large, heavy skillet with nonstick cooking spray, and place over medium-high heat. Melt 2 to 3 tablespoons of butter in it, and drop in the tuna mixture by the tablespoonful. Fry until brown, turn, and brown other side. It takes two batches to cook all of this mixture in my skillet; add the rest of the butter when you make the second batch. Serve with Easy Remoulade Sauce (see page 214), which takes all of 2 or 3 minutes to make.

Yield: 4 or 5 servings. Assuming 5 servings, and not including the Easy Remoulade Sauce, each will have 5 grams of carbohydrates and 1 gram of fiber, for a total of 4 grams of usable carbs and 32 grams of protein.

☉ Ginger Mustard Fish

4 fish fillets, about 6 ounces (175 g) each—tilapia, cod,
   orange roughy, what have you

4 tablespoons butter

2 teaspoons minced garlic or 4 cloves garlic, crushed

2 teaspoons grated gingerroot

2 teaspoons spicy brown or Dijon mustard

1 tablespoon water

In a large, heavy skillet, start sautéing the fish in the butter over medium-low heat; 4 to 5 minutes per side should be plenty. Remove the fish to a plate.

Add the garlic, gingerroot, mustard, and water to the skillet, and stir everything together well. Put the fish back in, turning it over once, carefully, to make sure both sides get acquainted with the sauce. Let it cook for another minute or so, then serve. Scrape the sauce out of the skillet over the fish.

Yield: 4 servings, each with 1 gram of carbohydrates, a trace of fiber, and 31 grams of protein.

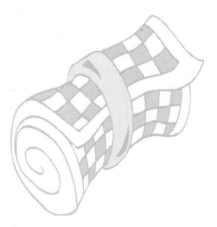

☺ Swordfish Veracruz

This is so simple and quick—yet it's the sort of thing you'd pay big bucks for at a fancy restaurant. Salsa verde is a green salsa made from tomatillos. Look for it in the Mexican or International section of your grocery store.

> 24 ounces swordfish steaks (700 g)
> 1/2 cup ruby red grapefruit juice—I like to use fresh-squeezed (100 ml)
> 1/2 teaspoon ground cumin
> 1 tablespoon oil
> 1/4 cup salsa verde (50 ml)

Cut the swordfish into 4 servings, and place on a plate with a rim. Mix together the grapefruit juice and the cumin, and pour it over the steaks, turning them to coat both sides. Let the swordfish steaks sit in the grapefruit juice for 5 minutes or so.

Spray a large, heavy skillet with nonstick cooking spray, and place over medium heat. When the skillet is hot, add the oil, and then the fish. Sauté for 4 minutes per side. Then pour in the grapefruit juice from the plate and let the fish cook in it for another minute or two, turning once.

Place the fish on serving plates, top each serving with a tablespoon of salsa verde, and serve.

Yield: 4 servings, each with 4 grams of carbohydrates, a trace of fiber, and 34 grams of protein.

Variation: You can expand this recipe a bit by serving the fish on a bed of avocado slices—split one avocado between the 4 servings—and sprinkling chopped fresh cilantro on top. This will take you up to 8 grams of carbohydrates per serving and 2 grams of fiber, for a total of 6 grams of usable carbs.

⊕ Truite au Bleu

This is more a method of preparation than a recipe, and it's a true classic. Expand or contract this recipe at will, to serve however many diners you have.

  Water

  Cider vinegar

  Bay leaves

  Peppercorns or coarse cracked pepper

  Salt or Vege-Sal

  Trout, cleaned and beheaded, but with the skin still on—about 10 ounces (300 g) per serving as a main course, or 5 or 6 ounces (150 g) per serving as a first course

  Butter

You'll need a pan big enough for the trout to lie flat—I generally do just one big trout, weighing about a pound (500 g), and the only pan I have where it can lie flat is my big soup kettle. Use what you have, but it should be a pan that won't react with acid—stainless steel, enamelware, anodized aluminum, or stove-top glassware.

Next you make up a solution of water and vinegar, just enough to completely cover the trout. The proportions you want are roughly 3 or 4 parts water to 1 part vinegar. I find that 1 1/2 quarts (1.5 l) of water and 1 1/2 cups (350 ml) of vinegar are about right for my pan. Pour this solution in your pan, and turn the burner to high. Stir in 1 or 2 bay leaves, 1/2 tablespoon (7 ml) of pepper per quart (litre), and 1 teaspoon (5 ml) of salt or Vege-Sal per quart (litre). Bring this mixture to a simmer.

Simply lower the trout into the simmering solution, turn the burner to medium-low, and let the fish simmer for about 5 minutes. Lift the fish carefully out of the simmering solution, and serve with a pitcher of melted butter to pour over the fish.

Yield: Servings will depend on how many fish you cook, of course. The fish itself is carb-free, and of course most of the poaching solution is discarded—you can figure on no more than a gram of carbohydrates per serving, no fiber, and 59 grams of protein in a 10-ounce (300 g) trout.

☉ Mock Lobster

Monkfish has long been known as "poor man's lobster," so I decided to play up the similarity. Your microwave is great for cooking fish, and as for quick, let's face it—if this dish cooked any faster, you'd go back in time. Feel free to double or triple this. You'll just need to use a bigger plate (a glass pie plate will work beautifully) and add just a minute or two extra cooking time.

> 1 ½ tablespoons butter
>
> 6 ounces monkfish fillet (175 g)
>
> Lemon wedges

Put the butter on a microwaveable plate. Nuke it for 30 seconds at 70 percent power, or until melted.

Place the monkfish in the butter and turn it over to coat both sides. Cover the fish with microwave-safe plastic wrap. Nuke for 1 ½ minutes at 50 percent power. Uncover the fish, turn it over, and recover with the plastic wrap. Nuke for 30 seconds more at 50 percent power. Let it stand for a minute (or, if you're making another serving, a minute or two more), remove the plastic wrap, and check for doneness. If necessary, re-cover and give it another 30 seconds or so, then serve with lemon wedges.

Yield: 1 serving, with only a trace of carbohydrates, no fiber, and 25 grams of protein.

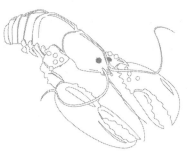

☉ Mock Lobster with Garlic

You'll notice a certain similarity to the previous recipe, but garlic changes the whole flavor.

> 1 1/2 tablespoons butter
>
> 1/2 teaspoon minced garlic or 1 clove garlic, crushed
>
> 6 ounces monkfish fillet (175 g)

Put the butter on a microwaveable plate. Nuke it for 30 seconds at 70 percent power, or until melted. Stir the garlic into the butter.

Place the monkfish in the butter and turn it over to coat both sides. Cover the fish with microwave-safe plastic wrap. Nuke for 1 1/2 minutes at 50 percent power. Uncover the fish, turn it over, and recover with the plastic wrap. Nuke for 30 seconds more at 50 percent power. Let it stand for a minute (or, if you're making another serving, a minute or two more), remove the plastic wrap, and check for doneness. If necessary, re-cover and give it another 30 seconds or so, then serve.

Yield: 1 serving, with only a trace of carbohydrates, no fiber, and 25 grams of protein.

⏱ Sea Bass with Tapenade Cream Sauce

Another one of those recipes that would impress the heck out of you at a restaurant but is very little trouble to make for yourself at home.

12 ounces sea bass fillet (350 g)

3 tablespoons olive oil

1/4 medium onion

1/2 teaspoon minced garlic or 1 clove garlic, crushed

2 tablespoons tapenade

1 tablespoon balsamic vinegar

1 teaspoon lemon juice

3 tablespoons heavy cream

Salt and pepper

If the bass is in one piece, cut it into two equal portions. Brush with 1 tablespoon of the olive oil, and put it under a broiler set on High, 3 or 4 inches (7 to 10 cm) from the heat. The length of time the fish will need to broil will depend on its thickness. I use fillets about 1 1/2 inch (4 cm) thick, and they take about 5 to 6 minutes per side.

While the fish is broiling, slice the quarter-onion in half lengthwise, and then slice as thinly as possible. Put the rest of the olive oil in a medium-size skillet over medium heat, and add the onion and garlic. Sauté together for 3 to 4 minutes. Add the tapenade, stir in, and sauté for a few more minutes. (Remember that somewhere in here you'll need to turn the fish!)

Now, stir the vinegar and lemon juice into the mixture in your skillet, and let it cook down for 1 to 2 minutes. Stir in the cream, and let the whole thing cook down for another minute.

When the fish is done, place it on two serving plates. Salt and pepper the sauce to taste, spoon over the fish, then serve.

Yield: 2 servings, each with 4 grams of carbohydrates, a trace of fiber, and 32 grams of protein.

☺ Jalapeño Lime Scallops

I served this as a first course at a little dinner party, and everyone agreed they'd never had a better scallop dish, even at a restaurant. A sterling example of how a few perfect ingredients can combine to make something greater than the sum of the parts. By the way, you can use sea scallops instead of bay scallops if you like, but since they're bigger, they'll take longer to cook.

> 4 tablespoons butter
>
> 1 1/2 pounds bay scallops (750 g)
>
> 2 medium-size fresh jalapeños
>
> 3 tablespoons lime juice
>
> 3 tablespoons chopped cilantro
>
> Guar or xanthan

Melt the butter in a big, heavy skillet over medium heat. Add the scallops and sauté for a few minutes, stirring often. In the meanwhile, split the jalapeños lengthwise and remove the stems, seeds, and ribs. Slice them lengthwise again, into quarters, then slice them as thin as you can crosswise. Add to the skillet, and sauté the jalapenos with the scallops until the scallops are cooked through—they should look quite opaque all over. (And wash your hands! You must always wash your hands after handling hot peppers, or you'll be sorry the next time you touch your eyes, lips, or nose.)

Stir in the lime juice, and cook for another minute while you chop the cilantro. Thicken the pan juices slightly with the guar or xanthan, and divide the scallops between serving plates, spooning the pan juices over them. Scatter the cilantro on top, and serve.

Yield: 4 main-dish servings or 6 first-course servings. Assuming 4 servings, each will have 6 grams of carbohydrates, a trace of fiber, and 29 grams of protein.

chapter six

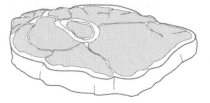

15~Minute Steaks and Chops

Steaks, chops, and other simple slabs of protein are classic fast low-carb fare, and let's face it, they're very nice simply broiled. But sometimes you want a little change. Here you'll find some quick-and-easy ways to add interest to these familiar foods.

⊕ Steak with Horseradish Butter

Horseradish is a classic accompaniment to beef.

> 1 steak, 12 to 16 ounces, well-marbled—sirloin, rib eye, strip steak, or the like (350 to 500 g)
> 2 tablespoons butter
> 1 to 2 teaspoons prepared horseradish
> Salt and pepper

Broil the steak as close to the flame as you can get it, with the broiler set on High. For a 1-inch-thick (2-cm-thick) steak, I like about 6 to 6 1/2 minutes per side, but you should experiment and cook it to your liking.

While the steak is broiling, put the butter and the horseradish in your food processor with the S-blade in place, or in your blender, and run just long enough to blend. When the steak is done cooking, salt and pepper it, divide it into servings, and scoop a dollop of the horseradish butter on each serving.

Yield: 2 or 3 servings. Each 6-ounce (170 g) serving will have no more than 1 gram of carbohydrates, no fiber, and 24 grams of protein.

> **Note:** Be careful when buying prepared horseradish! A lot of brands add sugar. Look for one that only contains grated horseradish root and vinegar. (I like Woeber's.)

⊕ Orange Steak

This gives a nice tang to a simple grilled steak.

    3 tablespoons orange juice
    1 tablespoon dry sherry
    1 teaspoon soy sauce
    1 teaspoon Splenda
    1/2 teaspoon minced garlic or 1/2 clove garlic, crushed
    12 to 16 ounces steak, 1/2 inch (1 cm) thick—rib eye, sirloin, strip steaks,
        anything tender and fit for broiling (350 to 500 g)
    Salt or Vege-Sal and pepper

Combine the orange juice, sherry, soy sauce, Splenda, and garlic. Put the steak on a plate, pour the orange juice mixture over it, and turn it over a few times to coat the whole surface. Let the steak sit for 2 to 3 minutes.

Now broil the steak as close as possible to a high flame until it's done to your liking—4 1/2 to 5 minutes per side is about right for me. Baste both sides with the orange mixture when you turn it! Salt, pepper, and serve.

Yield: The number of servings will depend on the size of your steak. Given a 12-ounce (350 g) steak, I'd call it 2 servings, each with 3 grams of carbohydrates, a trace of fiber, and 25 grams of protein.

☉ Costa Brava Steak

I was surprised that this traditional, anchovy-based Spanish sauce was not particularly fishy—just rich, mellow, and complex.

> 12 to 16 ounces steak, 1/2 to 3/4 inch thick (1 to 2 cm)—rib eye, sirloin,
>   strip, anything tender and fit for broiling (350 to 500 g)
> 1/3 cup shelled walnuts (30 g)
> 3 anchovy fillets
> 1/2 teaspoon red wine vinegar or sherry vinegar
> 1/3 cup olive oil (70 ml)

Start the steak broiling as close as possible to a high flame. Set your timer to remind you when to turn it—for a steak 1/2 inch thick (1 cm), 5 minutes per side is about right for my tastes.

While the steak is broiling, put the walnuts, anchovies, and vinegar in your food processor with the S-blade in place. Pulse to chop everything together—unless your machine is smaller than mine, the mixture will end up out against the walls of the processor bowl pretty quickly!

Scrape down the sides of the processor to get the mixture back into the path of the blade. Put the top back on, turn the processor on, and slowly pour in about half of the olive oil. If necessary, scrape down the sides of the processor again at this point, then turn it back on and add the rest of the oil.

When both sides of the steak are done, spread this sauce over the steak. Turn the broiler to Low, put the steak back under it for just a minute, then serve.

Yield: The number of servings will depend on the size of your steak. Assuming a 12-ounce (350 g) steak, I'd call it 2 servings, each with 3 grams of carbohydrates and 1 gram of fiber, for a total of 2 grams of usable carbs and 31 grams of protein.

☉ Inauthentic Bulgogi Steak

True Bulgogi is a popular Korean dish made with very thin sheets of sliced beef. We don't have time in our 15 minutes to carefully slice up our beef, so we're using good old steak, and boy, are the results spectacular!

¼ medium onion

2 teaspoons minced garlic or 4 cloves garlic, peeled

¼ cup soy sauce (50 ml)

2 tablespoons Splenda

1 teaspoon pepper

A few dashes Tabasco

2 tablespoons toasted sesame oil

1 ½ pounds tender, well-marbled steaks, 1/2 inch (1 cm)
   thick—sirloin, rib eye, strip, whatever you like (750 g)

Put the onion, garlic, soy sauce, Splenda, pepper, Tabasco, and sesame oil in a food processor with the S-blade in place, and run it until the onion is pulverized.

Place the steaks on a plate and pour the seasoning mixture over them, turning them so that they're coated on both sides. Let the steaks sit for a minute, then place them on a broiler rack. Broil the steaks as close to a high flame as possible until they're done to your liking—4 ½ to 5 minutes per side is right for me. When you're turning the steaks, spoon some of the seasoning mixture from the plate, first over the side that's already done, and then over the side about to be broiled.

Yield: 4 servings. Calculations show 4 grams per serving and a trace of fiber, but that would only be true if you ate all of the seasoning mixture, which you won't. Figure closer to 2 grams of carbs and 26 grams of protein.

☉ Steak Diane

This is actually a simplified version of a classic recipe—the original version didn't fit into our 15-minute time frame. It's really good, though!

> 12-ounce steak, 1/2 inch (1 cm) thick* (350 g)
>
> 2 tablespoons butter
>
> 3 scallions, finely minced
>
> 1 tablespoon minced parsley
>
> 1 1/2 teaspoons minced garlic
>
> 1 tablespoon brandy
>
> 2 tablespoons dry sherry
>
> 1 1/2 teaspoons Worcestershire sauce

* Use rib eye, sirloin, strip, or whatever you like.

In a heavy skillet over medium-high heat, sauté the steak in the butter—figure 5 to 6 minutes per side. While that's happening, mince up the scallions and parsley.

When the steak is done to your liking, remove it to a platter and keep it warm. Turn the burner down to medium. Add the scallions, parsley, and garlic, and sauté in the butter for a minute or so. Add the brandy, sherry, and Worcestershire sauce, turn the heat back up, and boil hard while stirring, to scrape any nice brown bits off the bottom of the pan. Let it boil for a minute or so to reduce, pour it over the steak, and serve.

Yield: 2 servings, each with 3 grams of carbohydrates and 2 grams of fiber, for a total of just 1 gram of usable carbs and 25 grams of protein.

☺ Many-Pepper Steak

This is so good! Make the Cumin Mushrooms as a side and toss some bagged salad with ranch or vinaigrette, and you're livin' large—without gettin' large!

> 12-ounce steak, 1/2 inch (1 cm) thick* (350 g)
>
> Many-Pepper Steak Seasoning (see page 218)

* I think rib eye is best for this, but it's not essential; use what you like.

Sprinkle both sides of the steak liberally with the Many-Pepper Steak Seasoning—about 1 teaspoon per side—and broil close to the flame until done to your liking (5 minutes per side is about right for me).

Yield: 2 servings, each with 3 grams of carbohydrates and 1 gram of fiber, for a total of 2 grams of usable carbs and 25 grams of protein.

About Lamb Steaks

Everybody's heard of lamb chops, but lamb steaks are harder to find. However, I think they're better and I can get them cheaper than most lamb chops, too. Here's how: I wait until whole legs of lamb are on sale at my grocery store—at least a few times a year they go as low as $1.99 a pound. When they do, I buy one or two, and have the meat guy at the grocery store slice a smallish roast off either end (these make far more sense for small households than a whole leg of lamb), and slice the center into steaks 1/2 inch (1 cm) thick. I've never been charged for this service. When I get them home, I bag everything up and stash it in the freezer—where they don't last very long, since I'm hopelessly devoted to lamb!

However, if you prefer, you can make any of these lamb recipes with 1/2-inch-thick (1-cm-thick) lamb chops, instead.

☺ Soy and Sesame Glazed Lamb Steaks

2 lamb steaks, 6 to 8 ounces (175 g) each, 1/2 inch (1 cm) thick

2 tablespoons olive oil

1 teaspoon minced garlic or 2 cloves garlic, crushed

2 scallions, minced

2 tablespoons soy sauce

1 teaspoon Splenda

6 drops or 1/4 teaspoon blackstrap molasses*

2 teaspoons sesame oil

* I keep my molasses in a squeeze container to make it easy to measure out very small quantities.

In a heavy skillet, start sautéing the lamb steaks in the oil over high heat. Cook for 5 to 6 minutes per side.

While the lamb is browning, prepare and combine the garlic, scallions, soy sauce, Splenda, molasses, and sesame oil.

Remove the lamb from the skillet, add the soy sauce mixture, and stir a bit. Replace the lamb in the skillet, turn it once to coat with sauce, and cook it for another 1 to 2 minutes per side. Serve, scraping the liquid from the pan over the lamb steaks.

Yield: 2 servings. Assuming each steak is 6 ounces (175 g), each will have 4 grams of carbohydrates and 1 gram of fiber, for a total of 3 grams of usable carbs and 23 grams of protein.

⏱ Curried Lamb Steak

    2 tablespoons butter

    2 teaspoons curry powder

    1 teaspoon minced garlic or 2 cloves garlic, crushed

    2 lamb steaks, 6 to 8 ounces (175 g) each, ¹/₂ inch (1 cm) thick

Melt the butter in large, heavy skillet over medium heat. Add the curry powder and garlic, stir, and add the lamb steak. Cover with a tilted lid and cook for 7 minutes. Turn, recover with a tilted lid, and cook for another 7 minutes. Remove the lamb to serving plates, scrape the curry butter over the steaks, and serve.

Yield: 2 servings. Assuming each steak is 6 ounces, each will have 2 grams of carbohydrates and 1 gram of fiber, for a total of 1 gram of usable carbs and 23 grams of protein.

⏱ Barbecued Lamb Steaks

    2 lamb steaks, 6 to 8 ounces each (175 g), ¹/₂ inch (1 cm) thick

    1 tablespoon plus 1 teaspoon sugar-free ketchup

    1 tablespoon plus 1 teaspoon cider vinegar

    1 tablespoon plus 1 teaspoon Worcestershire sauce

    1 teaspoon spicy brown mustard

Broil the lamb steaks close to the flame for 6 to 7 minutes. While the steaks are cooking, combine the ketchup, vinegar, Worcestershire sauce, and mustard.

Turn the steaks and broil the second side for 3 to 4 minutes. Spoon the sauce over the steaks and broil for another 2 to 3 minutes. Serve.

Yield: 2 servings. Assuming each steak is 6 ounces (175 g), each will have 4 grams of carbohydrates, a trace of fiber, and 23 grams of protein.

About Pork Loin

Whole pork loin is another largish cut of meat that often goes on sale at attractive prices. Again, if you buy a whole pork loin, the nice people behind the meat counter will be glad to cut it to your specifications. Keep in mind, however, that pork ages poorly in the freezer—use it up within two to three months, or it will taste nasty.

☺ Pineapple Glazed Pork Loin

You can double this recipe if you like, but if your skillet's the size of mine, you'll have to cook it in two batches—which, of course, takes twice the time.

> 3/4 pound boneless pork loin, cut about 1/2 inch (1 cm) thick* (350 g)
>
> 1 to 2 tablespoons olive oil (15 to 30 ml)
>
> 2 tablespoons canned, crushed pineapple in juice
>
> 2 teaspoons cider vinegar
>
> 2 teaspoons Splenda
>
> 1 teaspoon spicy brown or Dijon mustard
>
> 1/2 teaspoon soy sauce
>
> 1 teaspoon minced garlic or 2 cloves garlic, crushed

* Feel free to use thinish pork chops, instead.

First, pound the pork until it's about 1/4 inch (5 mm) thick. Heat the oil in a heavy skillet over medium-high heat, and sauté the pork, covering it with a tilted lid. Give it 4 to 5 minutes per side.

While the pork's browning, combine the pineapple, vinegar, Splenda, mustard, soy sauce, and garlic. When the pork is browned on both sides, add this mixture to the skillet. Turn the pork over once or twice to coat. Put the tilted lid back on the pan, and cook for 1 to 2 minutes, turn, recover, and give it another 1 to 2 minutes. Remove to serving plates, and scrape any remaining liquid from the pan over the pork before serving.

Yield: 2 servings, each with 4 grams of carbohydrates, a trace of fiber, and 22 grams of protein.

☺ Chili Lime Pork Strips

I didn't know where else in the book to put this, but it was too good and too versatile to leave out! Use the strips for a Chili Lime Pork Salad or a Chili Lime Pork Omelet, or just wrap them up in low-carb tortillas with a little salsa and sour cream.

> 1 pound boneless pork loin (500 g)
> 1 to 2 tablespoons oil
> 1 1/2 teaspoons chili powder
> 1 tablespoon lime juice

Slice the pork as thinly as you can into small strips (this is easier if the pork is half-frozen). Heat the oil in a large, heavy skillet over medium-high heat, and add the pork. Stir-fry the pork strips until they're nearly done—about 6 to 7 minutes—then stir in the chili powder and lime juice. Continue stirring and cooking for another 3 to 4 minutes. These strips keep well for a few days in a closed container in the fridge.

Yield: 4 servings, each with 1 gram of carbohydrates, a trace of fiber, and 23 grams of protein.

☉ Cherry Chops

An unusual sauce of tart cherries and a crunch of toasted almonds enhance these pork chops. Don't expect this sauce to be cherry-red, though, unless you add a drop or two of food coloring.

> 4 thin pork chops, about 18 ounces (500 g) total
>
> Salt and pepper
>
> 1 tablespoon olive oil
>
> 1/2 cup canned tart cherries in water (pie cherries) (50 g)
>
> 1 tablespoon wine vinegar
>
> 1/4 teaspoon dry mustard
>
> 1/8 teaspoon ground cloves
>
> 1 1/2 tablespoons Splenda
>
> 1/8 teaspoon guar or xanthan
>
> 1/3 cup slivered almonds (30g)
>
> 1/2 tablespoon butter

Salt and pepper the chops lightly on both sides and start browning them in the oil in a heavy skillet over medium-high heat. Give them about 5 minutes per side. While that's happening, put the cherries, vinegar, mustard, cloves, Splenda, and guar or xanthan in a blender, and purée the whole thing together. (If you'd prefer to keep the cherries whole, you could just mix everything together well. I like it puréed.)

It's time to turn the chops now! While the chops are browning on their second side, start browning the almonds in the butter in a small skillet over medium heat. Stir frequently so they don't burn; you just want a touch of gold. When the almonds are toasted, don't forget to turn off the heat, and if you have an electric stove, remove the pan from the burner.

When the second side of the chops is browned—again, about 5 minutes—pour the cherry sauce over them, turn the burner to medium-low, and cover the skillet with a tilted lid. Let the whole thing simmer for 5 minutes and serve. Scrape the sauce from the skillet over the chops, and top each with toasted almonds.

Yield: 4 servings, each with 6 grams of carbohydrates and 1 gram of fiber, for a total of 5 grams of usable carbs and 22 grams of protein.

☉ Gingersnap Pork

Okay, it doesn't really have gingersnaps in it, but it is sweet and spicy and good!

    4 thin pork chops, about 18 ounces (500 g) total

    1 tablespoon olive oil

    1/2 cup cider vinegar (100 ml)

    1/2 teaspoon pepper

    1/4 teaspoon ground cloves

    1 tablespoon tomato paste

    3 tablespoons Splenda

    2 teaspoons grated gingerroot

    2 teaspoons lemon juice

    1/2 teaspoon salt or Vege-Sal

    1/4 cup finely diced celery, including leaves (30g)

In a heavy skillet over medium-high heat, start browning the chops in the oil. While that's happening, put the vinegar, pepper, cloves, tomato paste, Splenda, gingerroot, lemon juice, and Vege-Sal in a blender, and run it for a second or two to blend.

When the chops are browned on both sides—about 5 minutes per side—pour the sauce over them, scatter the celery over the whole thing, turn the burner to low, and cover with a tilted lid. Let it simmer for 5 minutes, then serve. Don't forget to scrape the extra sauce out of the pan and over the chops!

Yield: 4 servings, each with 5 grams of carbohydrates, a trace of fiber, and 20 grams of protein.

About Pork Steaks

Shoulder steaks are my favorite cut of pork—I think they're juicier and more flavorful than pork loin or most chops, probably because they have more fat! Pork steaks have a lot of advantages for the low-carber in a hurry—they cook quickly, they're often quite cheap, and they take to a variety of easy seasonings, so you can vary them at will. Here are the two ways I most often cook pork steaks, plus a very slightly more complicated bonus recipe.

☉ Sautéed Pork Steak

Pork steaks vary considerably in size. Whether you have a single-serving pork steak or a two-serving pork steak will depend on the size of your steak, not to mention the size of your appetite. Feel free to do two steaks at a time if they'll fit in your skillet.

> Olive oil
>
> Pork shoulder steak, no more than 1/2 inch (1 cm) thick
>
> Sprinkle-on seasoning of your choice—Cajun, Creole, Soul, Barbecue,
>   and Jerk seasonings are all great used this way

Heat a heavy skillet over medium-high heat. Add the olive oil, slosh it around, and throw in the pork steak. Sprinkle the top with the sprinkle-on seasoning. Let the steak cook for about 7 minutes, or until it's well-browned and a bit crusty on the bottom. Flip it, sprinkle the seasoning on the cooked side, and let it cook for another 7 minutes, or until well-browned on the second side and cooked through. Serve.

Yield: How many servings this makes will depend—as noted—on how big your steak is. I can eat a medium-size pork steak all by myself, and I often do! The sprinkle-on seasoning is unlikely to add more than 1 gram of carbs per serving, but do read your labels and choose brands with little or no sugar, or make your own.

> **Note:** Instead of sprinkle-on seasoning, you can add some minced garlic toward the end, and flip the steak once or twice to flavor both sides. Don't add the garlic right at the beginning, though; it's liable to burn and go bitter on you.

☉ Grilled Pork Steak

Cooking your pork steaks in your electric tabletop grill cuts the cooking time down to 7 to 8 minutes. The trade-off is that your steak will be less browned and crusty than if you'd done it in a skillet.

> Pork shoulder steak, no more than 1/2 inch (1 cm) thick
>
> Sprinkle-on seasoning—Cajun, Creole, Soul, Barbecue, and Jerk seasonings are all good used this way

Preheat your electric tabletop grill.

While it's heating, lay the steak on a plate and sprinkle both sides liberally with the seasoning of your choice. When the grill is hot, throw the pork steak in and give it 7 to 8 minutes, or until it's cooked through. Serve.

Yield: Again, how many servings this makes depends on the size of your steak, but the carb count is unlikely to be more than 1 gram, even if you eat the whole thing.

☉ Pork Crusted Pork!

> 8-ounce pork shoulder steak, 1/2 inch (1 cm) thick (250 g)
>
> 1/3 cup crushed barbecue-flavor pork rinds (50 g)
>
> 1 to 2 tablespoons oil

Coat both sides of the pork steak with the crushed pork rinds. (It's easiest to spread the crushed pork rinds on a plate and press each side of the pork steak into them.) Heat the oil in a heavy skillet over medium-high heat, and sauté the steak until it's crisp on both sides and cooked through—about 7 minutes per side.

Yield: 1 or 2 servings. There are no carbohydrates or fiber here at all, and the whole steak will have about 45 grams of protein.

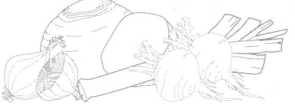

chapter seven

15~Minute Main Dish Salads

Main dish salads are one of the greatest ways to eat low carb. They're quick, simple, delicious, beautiful to look at, offer endless variety, and pack more nutrition into a single meal than most anything else you can think of. I hope you'll serve these main dish salads often, especially on hot summer days— and nights.

Here are some new ideas to take you beyond your old standby tuna salad and the ubiquitous chicken Caesar.

☉ Vietnamese Chicken Salad

I tried making a really authentic Vietnamese Chicken Salad, and it was delicious—but it also took forever to make—including an hour and a half to poach a whole chicken! I was determined to streamline the process so you could enjoy this wonderful treat. Here it is.

> 1 pound boneless, skinless chicken breast or precooked chicken
> breast slices (500 g)
> 6 cups bagged coleslaw mix (500 g)
> 4 scallions
> 1 batch Nuoc Cham (see page 214)
> 1 ruby red grapefruit
> 2 tablespoons sesame seeds
> 2 tablespoons chopped fresh mint
> 2 tablespoons chopped fresh cilantro

If you're starting with raw chicken breasts, you'll want to start cooking them first. I do mine for about 6 minutes in my electric tabletop grill, but you could sauté them, if you prefer. If you're sautéing them, you may want to take a minute to pound them thin so they cook through within our 15-minute time limit. If you're really in a hurry, feel free to use precooked chicken breast slices instead, although you'll pay a premium for them.

Put the bagged coleslaw mix in a bowl, and slice the scallions into it. Make the Nuoc Cham—this is very quick to do—pour it over the cabbage, and toss well. Set aside.

Cut the grapefruit in half, and loosen the sections by running the tip of a knife around each one.

Put the sesame seeds in a small, dry skillet, and shake them over a high flame for about 2 minutes, or until they start to jump around in the pan and make popping sounds. Turn off the burner and set the pan aside.

Okay, the chicken is ready now! If you're using unsliced breasts, put them on a cutting board and thinly slice them.

Now, toss the cabbage one more time to make sure the dressing is evenly distributed. Mound it on 4 serving plates. Top each serving with sliced chicken. Spoon 1/4 of the grapefruit sections around each portion. Scatter 1 tablespoon each of chopped mint and chopped cilantro over each serving (or easier yet, use kitchen shears to snip the herbs directly onto each serving), scatter 1/2 tablespoon of sesame seeds over each plate, and serve.

Yield: 4 generous servings, each with 18 grams of carbohydrates and 5 grams of fiber, for a total of 13 grams of usable carbs (virtually all of them from vegetables!) and 30 grams of protein.

✳ This has less than 250 calories, too!

☺ Tuna Salad with Lemon and Capers

I've always loved the bright, sunny flavors of lemon and capers in foods cooked "piccata." This is my way of adding those Mediterranean flavors to tuna salad.

> 5-ounce can tuna, drained (150 g)
>
> ¹/₂ cup diced sweet red onion (50 g)
>
> 2 stalks celery, diced
>
> ¹/₃ cup chopped parsley (30 g)
>
> 1 tablespoon capers
>
> 1 tablespoon lemon juice
>
> 1 tablespoon olive oil
>
> 1 tablespoon mayonnaise

Just drain the tuna, put it in a bowl with the onion, celery, parsley, and capers, and mix. Add the lemon juice, olive oil, and mayonnaise, and stir it together until it's thoroughly combined. It's nice to serve this on a bed of lettuce, but it's not essential.

Yield: 2 servings, each with 5 grams of carbohydrates and 2 grams of fiber, for a total of 3 grams of usable carbs and 19 grams of protein.

❀ Only 214 calories per serving!(If you use water packed tuna.)

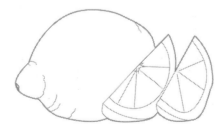

⊕ Curried Tuna Salad

Good as-is, or as an omelet filling (see page 34).

> 1/2 cup slivered almonds (60 g)
>
> 2 tablespoons plus 1/2 teaspoon butter
>
> 1 large stalk celery, diced
>
> 1 scallion, sliced
>
> 6-ounce can tuna, drained (175 g)
>
> 2 tablespoons sour cream
>
> 2 tablespoons mayonnaise
>
> 1 tablespoon lemon juice
>
> 1/8 teaspoon pepper
>
> 3/4 teaspoon curry powder

Sauté the almonds in 2 tablespoons of butter over medium-high heat, stirring frequently, until the almonds are golden. Remove from the heat and set aside.

Dice the celery and slice the scallion, open and drain the tuna, and combine them all in a mixing bowl. Add the sour cream, mayo, lemon juice, and pepper.

In your smallest skillet, melt the last 1/2 teaspoon of butter and sauté the curry powder in it, over medium heat, for just a minute (this brings out the full flavor of the curry). Scrape the curry butter into the salad, and mix until the curry is well-distributed throughout. Stir in the almonds, and serve.

Yield: If you serve this as a salad—over a bed of greens is nice—this makes 2 servings, each with 6 grams of carbohydrates and 2 grams of fiber, for a total of 4 grams of usable carbs and 22 grams of protein.

☻ Tuna "Rice" Salad

Can you tell I like tuna?

¹/₂ head cauliflower

5-ounce can tuna (150 g)

2 tablespoons lime juice

2 ¹/₂-ounce can sliced ripe olives, drained (75 g)

14-ounce can quartered artichoke hearts, drained (500 g)

¹/₂ cup mayonnaise (100 ml)

1 teaspoon dried dill weed

Run the cauliflower through the shredding blade of your food processor. Put it in a microwaveable casserole with a lid, add a couple of tablespoons of water, cover, and nuke on High for 7 minutes.

While that's happening, combine the tuna, lime juice, olives, artichoke hearts, mayonnaise, and dill. When the cauliflower is done, pull it out of the microwave, drain it, and toss it in with everything else.

Obviously, if you don't like a warm salad, you'll have to chill this—but that takes more than 15 minutes! And it sure tastes good warm. If you really want it cooled quickly, you could put the cauliflower "rice" in a strainer and run cold water over it for a minute.

Yield: 3 servings, each with 12 grams of carbohydrates and 1 gram of fiber, for a total of 11 grams of usable carbs and 16 grams of protein.

☺ San Diego Tuna Salad

Yes, you really can get all of this—including the Guacamole Dressing—done in 15 minutes!

    1 batch Guacamole Dressing (see page 216)

    12 cups bagged mixed greens (1 kg)

    2/3 cup sliced ripe olives (70 g)

    1/2 cup diced sweet red onion (50 g)

    1 cup sliced mushrooms (100 g)

    8 tablespoons chopped cilantro

    8 tablespoons alfalfa sprouts

    Three 5-ounce cans tuna, drained (450 g)

    2 small tomatoes, cut into thin wedges

Make the Guacamole Dressing first.

In a large salad bowl, combine the mixed greens, olives, onion, mushrooms, cilantro and sprouts. Pour on the Guacamole Dressing, and toss thoroughly.

Pile the salad on 4 or 5 serving plates. Top each serving with drained tuna and decorate each serving with tomato wedges. Serve.

Yield: 4 or 5 servings. Assuming 5 servings, each will have 14 grams of carbohydrates and 6 grams of fiber, for a total of 8 grams of usable carbs and 27 grams of protein.

✻ This salad also contains 1059 milligrams of potassium and less than 350 calories. (If you use water packed tuna.)

☉ Crabamole Salad

Even if you're making the Guacamole Dressing right then, this is incredibly quick and easy. Feel free to substitute the seafood of your choice for the crab—flaked, cooked lobster or small salad shrimp would work well. Just don't use fake seafood, such as "Delicaseas"—the stuff has a whole pile of added carbs.

> 24 ounces bagged mixed greens (700 g)
> 1 pound cooked lump crabmeat (500 g)
> 1 batch Guacamole Dressing (see page 216)
> 16 cherry tomatoes

Arrange the mixed greens on 4 serving plates. Top each with crabmeat, then top that with the Guacamole Dressing, letting it run artistically down onto the greens. Cut the cherry tomatoes in half and arrange them around each portion. Serve.

Yield: 4 servings, each with 17 grams of carbohydrates and 8 grams of fiber, for a total of 9 grams of usable carbs and 28 grams of protein.

❋ There's also 1479 milligrams of potassium and 344 milligrams of calcium in each serving of this salad!

⊕ Border Town Chicken Salad

If you don't have any leftover cooked chicken around the house, feel free to use canned, chunk chicken. It's not the same, but it's still good. Or you could cut up purchased, precooked chicken breast slices.

    2 cups diced, cooked chicken (200 g)
    3 stalks celery, diced
    3 tablespoons chopped ripe olives
    3 tablespoons chopped cilantro
    1 batch Guacamole Dressing (see page 216)
    6 scallions, sliced

Just chop everything up, make the dressing, combine it all, and toss. You can serve this on a bed of lettuce, if you like, but I've been known to eat mine straight out of the mixing bowl.

Yield: 4 servings, each with 9 grams of carbohydrates and 3 grams of fiber, for a total of 6 grams of usable carbs and 24 grams of protein.

※ This salad is healthy, offering 720 milligrams of potassium and meaningful doses of calcium, vitamin A, and folic acid.

⊕ Smoked Salmon and Blue Cheese Salad

This salad is super easy, but elegant enough for an alfresco summer company lunch. It's also very simple to double or even triple.

    1 pound bagged romaine mix (500 g)
    1/3 cup bottled Dijon vinaigrette dressing (70 ml)
    8 ounces smoked salmon, flaked (250 g)
    3/4 cup crumbled blue cheese (30 g)
    6 scallions, sliced
    1/4 cup chopped Smokehouse almonds (30 g)

Put the romaine mix in a big salad bowl, and toss well with the dressing. Pile the greens on 3 plates, and top with the salmon, blue cheese, scallions, and almonds, in that order, then serve.

Yield: 3 servings, each with 10 grams of carbohydrates and 5 grams of fiber, for a total of 5 grams of usable carbs and 26 grams of protein.

☺ Ham-Pecan Salad with Apricot Dressing

Always read the labels and buy the lowest-sugar ham you can find—they vary quite a lot in carbohydrate content. This recipe assumes ham with 1 gram per 3 ounce (7 g) serving.

> 5 ounces cooked ham, diced (150 g)
>
> 1 stalk celery, diced
>
> 2 tablespoons diced red onion
>
> 1/4 cup chopped pecans (30 g)
>
> 2 tablespoons mayonnaise
>
> 2 teaspoons low-sugar apricot preserves
>
> 1 teaspoon spicy brown or Dijon mustard
>
> 1/4 teaspoon soy sauce

Mix together the ham, celery, onion, and pecans in a mixing bowl. Combine the mayonnaise, preserves, mustard, and soy sauce, and pour this over the ham mixture. Mix well, and serve. This is really nice on a bed of lettuce.

Yield: 1 serving, with 15 grams of carbohydrates and 4 grams of fiber, for a total of 11 grams of usable carbs and 29 grams of protein.

⊕ Satay Salad

Satay are little skewers of chicken or meat served with peanut sauce. This salad is quicker and easier than satay, and it turns what is usually an appetizer into a meal. This is also good if you substitute turkey tenderloins for the chicken breast. The 15-minute time on this recipe assumes that you've got Dana's Chicken Seasoning on hand—which, if you eat a lot of poultry, you should!

18 ounces boneless, skinless chicken breast (500 g)

Dana's Chicken Seasoning (see page 219)

1/3 cup rice vinegar (70 ml)

3 tablespoons natural peanut butter

2 tablespoons Splenda

2 tablespoons oil

3/4 teaspoon grated gingerroot

2 tablespoons toasted sesame oil

1 tablespoon soy sauce

3 tablespoons chopped dry-roasted peanuts

6 cups bagged romaine mix (500 g)

1 cup bagged coleslaw mix (70 g)

6 tablespoons chopped cilantro

3/4 cup bean sprouts (50 g)

Preheat your electric tabletop grill.

Sprinkle both sides of the chicken breasts with Dana's Chicken Seasoning, and slap 'em on the grill. Cook for 5 to 6 minutes, or until cooked through.

While the chicken's grilling, put the vinegar, peanut butter, Splenda, oil, gingerroot, sesame oil, and soy sauce in a blender, and run it for 10 to 20 seconds, scraping down the sides if needed. This is your dressing. Chop the peanuts while it's blending.

Assemble the romaine mix, coleslaw mix, cilantro, and bean sprouts in a large salad bowl. Pour the dressing over it, and toss thoroughly. Divide between 3 serving plates.

By now the chicken should be done. Pull it out of the grill, and slice each breast into thin strips. Divide the chicken between the 3 salads. Top each serving with 1 tablespoon of chopped peanuts, and serve.

Yield: 3 servings, each with 14 grams of carbohydrates and 5 grams of fiber, for a total of 9 grams of usable carbs and 48 grams of protein.

✳ You'll also get 880 milligrams of potassium in each serving!

☺ Debbie's Tuna-Cottage Cheese Scoops

My friend Debbie told me that she loved tuna mixed with cottage cheese, and "lots and lots of chopped dill pickles." So I tried it, and it made a really nice, simple lunch. This would travel well in a snap-top container, along with a baggie full of vegetables for scooping.

> 5-ounce can tuna, drained (150 g)
> 1/2 cup small-curd cottage cheese (100 g))
> 1/4 cup chopped dill pickle (30 g)
> 1/4 cup diced sweet red onion (30 g)
> 1 tablespoon mayonnaise
> Celery sticks, pepper strips, and/or cucumber rounds

Simply mix together the tuna, cottage cheese, dill pickle, red onion, and mayonnaise. Refrigerate until you're ready to eat it, and then scoop the tuna-cottage cheese salad up with the veggies!

Yield: 2 servings. Exclusive of the vegetables used for scooping, each serving will have 5 grams of carbohydrates and 1 gram of fiber, for a total of 4 grams of usable carbs and 26 grams of protein.

☺ Not-Quite-Middle-Eastern Salad Plus

Add protein to this fabulous side dish salad and it becomes a very posh summer lunch or supper.

>   1 batch Not-Quite-Middle-Eastern Salad (see page 180)
>   1 pound cooked crabmeat, lobster, or tiny shrimp (500 g)

Make the salad according to the instructions, then toss in the shellfish. Serve on a bed of lettuce.

Yield: 4 servings, each with 7 grams of carbohydrates and 3 grams of fiber, for a total of 4 grams of usable carbs and 22 grams of protein.

☺ Shrimp and Spinach Caesar Salad

Traditionally, Caesar Salad is made with romaine, but raw spinach is delicious, fabulous for you, and makes a pretty contrast with the shrimp and the eggs. If you don't have hard-boiled eggs on hand in the refrigerator, feel free to leave them out. (But why don't you have hard-boiled eggs on hand in the refrigerator?)

>   1 pound bagged, triple-washed baby spinach leaves (500 g)
>   1/3 cup bottled Caesar dressing (70 ml)
>   8 ounces cooked, peeled, bitsy little shrimp, either canned (drain first)
>   or frozen (thaw them!) (250 g)
>   2 hard-boiled eggs
>   3 tablespoons shredded parmesan cheese

Place the spinach in a big salad bowl, pour the dressing over it, and toss with reckless abandon until every square millimeter of every leaf is coated. Pile the spinach on 3 serving plates.

Divide the shrimp between the 3 plates, piling them in the middles of the beds of spinach.

Peel and slice the eggs, and arrange the slices around each pile of shrimp. Scatter 1 tablespoon of parmesan over each salad, and serve.

Yield: 3 servings, each with 7 grams of carbohydrates and 3 grams of fiber, for a total of 4 grams of usable carbs and 27 grams of protein.

✴ You'll also get 238 milligrams of calcium and a whopping 821 milligrams of potassium!

☺ Warm Chicken Liver Salad

You will like this if you like chicken livers, and you won't like it if you don't. Mmmmm. Chicken livers…

> 6 large chicken livers
>
> 2 tablespoons olive oil
>
> Salt or Vege-Sal and pepper
>
> 8 ounces bagged mixed greens—European or Parisian blends are good (250 g)
>
> 1/2 ripe avocado
>
> 1-inch (2 cm) wedge of a large sweet red onion, sliced paper thin
>
> 1/3 cup bottled Dijon vinaigrette (70 ml)

Cut each chicken liver into 3 or 4 pieces. Spray a large, heavy skillet with nonstick cooking spray and put it over medium-high heat. Add the oil and the livers. Sauté the livers, turning them frequently, until juices run clear and no pink spots show on the outsides. (Take care not to overcook the livers! They get tough if you overcook them.) Turn off the burner when they're done, and if you have an electric stove, remove the pan from the warm element. Salt and pepper lightly.

Pour the bagged greens into a big salad bowl. Use the tip of a spoon to scoop bits of avocado out of the shell and into the salad bowl. Add the sliced onion, pour the dressing over it all, and toss well. Divide the salad mixture between 2 plates.

Top each salad with half of the livers, and serve.

Yield: 2 servings, each with 15 grams of carbohydrates and 6 grams of fiber, for a total of 9 grams of usable carbs and 21 grams of protein.

✴ This recipe is truly healthy. It gives you 892 milligrams of potassium and well over your daily requirement for vitamin A, vitamin C, vitamin B2, vitamin B12, and folacin, not to mention half of your daily requirement for niacin, B6, and iron, and good doses of calcium, zinc, and B1. Indeed, I toyed with the idea of calling this "Big Pile of Nutrition Salad." It's got to be the most nutritious recipe in the book.

☉ Thai-Style Crab Salad in Avocados

Short on time, I got my pal Julie McIntosh to try out this recipe for me. She loved it the way I'd conceived of it, but suggested a little more cilantro, plus a little scallion, so that's what we did. Thanks, Julie!

1 ripe avocado

3 tablespoons lime juice

6-ounce can crabmeat, or 6 ounces cooked lump crabmeat (170 g)

1 teaspoon lemon juice

1/4 cup mayonnaise (50 ml)

2 tablespoons chopped cilantro

1 scallion, thinly sliced

1/4 teaspoon pepper, or to taste

Salt, if desired

Split the avocado in half, remove the seed, and sprinkle the cut surfaces with 1 tablespoon of the lime juice to prevent browning.

Combine the crabmeat, remaining lemon juice, mayonnaise, cilantro, scallion, pepper, and salt in a mixing bowl, and mix well. Stuff into the avocado halves, piling it high. Garnish with extra cilantro, if desired, and serve.

Yield: 2 servings, each with 9 grams of carbohydrates and 5 grams of fiber, for a total of 4 grams of usable carbs and 20 grams of protein.

※ This salad also provides 932 milligrams of potassium and 110 milligrams of calcium.

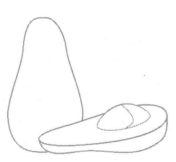

☺ Egg Salad Francais

Completely different from any egg salad you've ever had, and quite wonderful! This is actually a French tradition.

> 8 ounces bagged European style salad* (250 g)
>
> 2 scallions, sliced
>
> 1/3 cup bottled balsamic vinaigrette—I like Paul Newman's (70 ml)
>
> Salt and pepper
>
> 1/4 cup shredded Parmesan cheese** (30 g)
>
> 1 tablespoon vinegar
>
> 4 very fresh eggs

* The mixture should include some frizee, so read the label! If you can't find one with frizee, you can still make the salad, but it will be less authentic.

** It is very important to use good-quality shredded (not grated) Parmesan with no additives. Regular Parmesan in the round green shaker won't work; the cellulose in it messes it up for this.

First put 1 inch (2 cm) of water in a largish saucepan and put it over a burner set to medium-high. Ignore that for a minute while you put the greens and scallions in a big salad bowl. Pour the vinaigrette over the whole thing, add salt and pepper as desired, and toss well. Set aside.

Spray a microwaveable plate with nonstick cooking spray, and spread the Parmesan on it. Microwave on High for 1 minute.

While the cheese is nuking, let's get back to that water. It should be good and hot by now; turn it down to barely a simmer, add a tablespoon of vinegar, and poach the eggs in it. It helps to break each egg into a small cup or dish first, to make sure that it's good and fresh and that the yolk doesn't break. (If it does, keep it for something else and use another egg for poaching.) Then slide each egg gently into the water, and poach to the desired degree of doneness.

While the eggs are poaching, remove the Parmesan from the microwave—it will now be a crispy, lacy sheet. Break it up. Pile the salad on 2 serving plates and top each one with crispy Parmesan bits. Lift the now-poached eggs out of the pan with a slotted spoon, place 2 on each salad, and serve.

Yield: 2 servings, each with 10 grams of carbohydrates and 4 grams of fiber, for a total of 6 grams of usable carbs and 20 grams of protein.

⊕ Italian Roast Beef Salad

What a great meal, all from deli roast beef! Feel free to use leftover steak in this instead, should you happen to have any.

   2 quarts bagged European or Italian blend greens (750 g)

   ¼ cup thinly sliced sweet red onion (30 g)

   ¼ medium green pepper, sliced into small strips

   3 tablespoons extra virgin olive oil

   ½ teaspoon minced garlic or 1 clove garlic, crushed

   1 ½ tablespoons balsamic vinegar

   ½ teaspoon spicy brown or Dijon mustard

   ¼ cup crumbled Gorgonzola (30 g)

   4 ounces sliced deli roast beef (120 g)

   2 tablespoons toasted pine nuts

Place the greens, onion, and green pepper in a large salad bowl. Combine the oil and garlic, pour over the salad, and toss well. Stir together the balsamic vinegar and mustard, and set them aside.

Crumble the Gorgonzola (if you didn't buy it precrumbled), and add it to the salad. Slice the roast beef into strips, and throw it in there, too. Pour the balsamic vinegar mixture over the whole thing, and toss very well. Pile onto 2 serving plates, top each with a tablespoon of pine nuts, and serve.

Yield: 2 servings, each with 19 grams of carbohydrates and 9 grams of fiber, for a total of 10 grams of usable carbs and 27 grams of protein.

   ✻ You'll also get 1,153 milligrams of potassium and 247 milligrams of calcium, plus almost three times your daily requirements of vitamins C and A, and 100 percent of your daily requirement of folacin.

Note: Gorgonzola is the Italian version of blue cheese, a bit milder and creamier than most blue cheeses. If you can't find it, substitute any blue cheese you like.

☉ Aladdin Salad

I thought I was done with this chapter. Then I went to the Aladdin Restaurant in San Diego and had this fantastic salad. It was easy to duplicate, and way too good to leave out! If you're ever in San Diego, I highly recommend that you go to the Aladdin, by the way. I was very disappointed not to get back there before I left for home.

Salt and pepper

8 ounces boneless, skinless chicken breast (250 g)

8 cups romaine, broken up (600 g)

8 tablespoons chopped fresh cilantro

1/4 cup thinly sliced sweet red onion (30 g)

1/3 cup bottled balsamic vinaigrette—I like Paul Newman's (70 ml)

1/2 cup crumbled feta (50 g)

1/3 cup shelled pistachios* (50 g)

1 medium ripe tomato

* Look for these at Mediterranean or Middle Eastern groceries, or at a health food store with a good bulk section.

Preheat your electric tabletop grill while you salt and pepper the chicken lightly. Throw it on the grill, and set a timer for 6 minutes or so.

While the chicken's cooking, put the romaine, cilantro, and onion in a large salad bowl, pour on the dressing, and toss well. Pile this mixture on 2 serving plates. Scatter the feta and pistachios over the greens.

When the chicken is done, slice it into strips and divide it between the 2 salads. Slice the tomato into eighths, arrange 4 slices around each salad, then serve.

Yield: 2 large servings, each with 18 grams of carbohydrates and 7 grams of fiber, for a total of 11 grams of usable carbs and 40 grams of protein.

✻ You'll also get 1,333 milligrams of potassium and 320 milligrams of calcium!

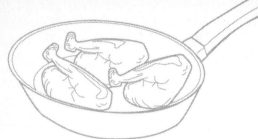

chapter eight

15-Minute Skillet Suppers

One-dish skillet meals are quick, versatile, and—since they generally contain both your protein and your vegetable—they eliminate the need to cook anything else. Furthermore, there's only one pan to wash!

Some of these "skillet suppers" can also be cooked in a wok. Use whatever you have.

⏱ Asian Pork and Cabbage

I know of few dishes that offer so much flavor for so little work.

> 1 pound boneless pork loin (500 g)
>
> 1/2 head cabbage
>
> 1 small onion
>
> Canola or peanut oil for stir-frying
>
> 1 tablespoon black bean sauce
>
> 1 to 2 tablespoons chili garlic paste

Slice the pork loin as thin as you possibly can—this is easier if the pork is partially frozen. Slice the cabbage about 1/2 inch (1 cm) thick, and cut across it a few times. Thinly slice the onion.

In a wok or large skillet, heat 3 to 4 tablespoons of oil over highest heat. As soon as it's hot, add the pork and stir-fry for 3 to 5 minutes. Add the cabbage and the onion, and continue stir-frying until the cabbage and onion are just tender-crisp. Stir in the black bean sauce and the chili garlic paste, and serve.

Yield: 3 servings, each with 6 grams of carbohydrates and 1 gram of fiber, for a total of 5 grams of usable carbs and 32 grams of protein.

> **Note:** Find Black Bean Sauce, an Asian condiment, in Asian or International grocery stores, or in the Asian section of larger grocery stores. I actually bought mine in the International aisle of Bloomingfoods, my beloved health food store. This has some sugar in it, but the amount of flavor it offers for the few carbs it adds is well worth it, to my mind. It keeps well in the fridge, so don't think you have to use it all up quickly.

⊕ Balsamic Lamb Skillet

Rich, different, and good!

> 1 pound lamb leg or shoulder, thinly sliced and cut into strips (500 g)
>
> 1/2 teaspoon minced garlic or 1 clove garlic, crushed
>
> 1/2 medium onion, sliced
>
> 1/4 cup olive oil (50 ml)
>
> 1/2 red bell pepper, sliced into small strips
>
> 1-pound bag triple-washed fresh spinach (500 g)
>
> 1/4 cup balsamic vinegar (50 ml)
>
> Salt and pepper
>
> Guar or xanthan
>
> 4 tablespoons toasted pine nuts

Over high heat, start sautéing the lamb, garlic, and onion in the olive oil. When the pinkness has faded from the lamb, add the red bell pepper, and stir that in, too.

When the lamb is cooked through and the onion is limp, add the spinach. You may have to add it in two or three batches to keep it from overwhelming your skillet, but it wilts quite quickly. Stir until the spinach is just barely limp. Don't overcook!

Stir in the balsamic vinegar, salt and pepper to taste (I like plenty of pepper in this), and thicken the pan juices with a sprinkle of guar or xanthan, if desired. Serve, and top each serving with a tablespoon of toasted pine nuts.

Yield: 4 servings, each with 9 grams of carbohydrates and 4 grams of fiber, for a total of 5 grams of usable carbs and 20 grams of protein.

☉ Chicken Skillet Alfredo

Who doesn't love Alfredo sauce?

> 1 1/2 pounds boneless, skinless chicken breast (750 g)
>
> 1/2 medium onion
>
> 3 tablespoons olive oil
>
> 1-pound bag frozen mixed cauliflower and broccoli (500 g) or 1/2 pound
>   frozen broccoli florets and 1/2 pound frozen cauliflowerets (250 g each)
>
> 1 cup jarred Alfredo sauce (250 ml)

Cut the chicken into 1-inch (2-cm) cubes, and slice your onion. Sauté the chicken and onion in the olive oil over medium heat.

While the chicken and onion are cooking, put the cauliflower and broccoli in a microwaveable casserole. Add a tablespoon or two of water, cover, and nuke it on High for 7 minutes. Go back and stir the chicken and onion while the veggies are nuking.

When the microwave goes "ding," check to see if the veggies are tender but not mushy. If they need a couple more minutes, give it to them. When the broccoli and cauliflower are done, drain them and add them to the skillet. Stir in the Alfredo sauce, heat through, and serve. Pass a little Parmesan to sprinkle on top, if you like.

Yield: 5 servings, each with 8 grams of carbohydrates and 3 grams of fiber, for a total of 5 grams of usable carbs and 35 grams of protein.

⊕ Chicken Skillet Roma

1 1/2 pounds boneless, skinless chicken breast, cut into 1-inch (2-cm) cubes (750 g)

1/2 green pepper, cut into small strips

1 small onion, sliced

2 cloves garlic, crushed, or 1 teaspoon minced garlic

3 tablespoons olive oil

2 1/4-ounce can sliced ripe olives, drained (50 g)

1 cup no-sugar-added spaghetti sauce (250 ml)

1/4 cup grated Parmesan cheese (30 g)

Sauté the chicken, pepper, onion, and garlic in the olive oil over medium-high heat. When all the pink is gone from the chicken, stir in the olives and spaghetti sauce, bring it to a simmer, and let it cook for just another minute. Serve with the Parmesan cheese on top.

Yield: 5 servings, each with 8 grams of carbohydrates and 2 grams of fiber, for a total of 6 grams of usable carbs and 33 grams of protein.

⊕ Italian Sausage with Onions and Peppers

Mmmmmmm! Like revisiting my childhood in the New York City area!

> 1 1/4 to 1 1/2 pounds Italian sausage links, hot or mild (625 to 750 g)
>
> 1/4 cup olive oil (50 ml)
>
> 1 1/2 large green peppers
>
> 1 large onion
>
> 1 clove garlic

Slice the sausage diagonally into 1/2-inch (1-cm) pieces, and sauté it in the olive oil over medium-high heat. Meanwhile, slice the peppers into medium-size strips, and slice the onion about 1/4 inch (5 mm) thick. When the sausage is about half done, stir in the peppers, onion, and garlic. Cook until the sausage is well done and the onion is limp and translucent. Serve.

Yield: 4 servings, each with 7 grams of carbohydrates and 1 gram of fiber, for a total of 6 grams of usable carbs and 21 grams of protein.

⊕ Italian Sausage with Onions, Peppers, Tomato Sauce, and Cheese

Make the Italian Sausage with Onions and Peppers as described above. When it's done, stir in:

> 1 cup no-sugar-added spaghetti sauce (250 ml)

Then top with:

> 1 cup (100 g) shredded mozzarella cheese

Cover the skillet for a couple of minutes to let the sauce heat through and the cheese melt. Serve.

Yield: 4 servings, each with 12 grams of carbohydrates and 3 grams of fiber, for a total of 9 grams of usable carbs and 28 grams of protein.

> **Note:** One of the lowest carbohydrate nationally distributed spaghetti sauces is Hunt's Original Style No Sugar Added. (They also make an Original Style with sugar, so read the label!) Each 1/2-cup (120 ml) serving contains 9 grams of carbohydrates and 3 grams of fiber, for a total of 6 grams of usable carbs. I really like this stuff!

☺ New-Fangled Farm Fry

In Peg Bracken's classic cookbook, *The I Hate To Cook Book*, there was a recipe for eggs cooked with potatoes, onions, and cheese, called "Old Fashioned Farm Fry." Here's my low-carb, twenty-first century version.

4 slices bacon

1 cup cauliflowerets, chopped into 1/2-inch (1-cm) pieces (150 g)

1 cup diced turnip, chopped into 1/2-inch (1-cm) pieces (150 g)

1/2 cup diced onion (50 g)

4 eggs

1/2 cup shredded cheddar cheese (50 g)

Salt and pepper

Chop the bacon up into smallish bits—kitchen shears are good for this. Start the bacon cooking in a big skillet. Combine the cauliflowerets and turnip in a microwaveable dish, add a couple of tablespoons of water, cover, and microwave on High for 7 minutes.

Drain the vegetables when they're done. Drain all but a few tablespoons of fat off the bacon, and add the cauliflower, turnip, and onion to the skillet. Sauté until the onion is translucent. Scramble the eggs with a fork, pour them into the skillet, sprinkle the cheese over the whole thing, and stir until the eggs are set. Salt and pepper to taste, and serve.

Yield: 2 servings, each with 12 grams of carbohydrates and 3 grams of fiber, for a total of 9 grams of usable carbs and 24 grams of protein.

⊕ Shrimp and Mushroom Sauté

Quick and easy enough for the family, yet impressive enough for company!

> 2 tablespoons olive oil
>
> 2 tablespoons butter
>
> 8 ounces sliced mushrooms (250 g)
>
> 1/2 medium onion
>
> 1 pound cleaned, shelled shrimp (500 g)
>
> 1/2 teaspoon minced garlic or 1 clove garlic, crushed
>
> 1 tablespoon lemon juice
>
> 1 tablespoon dry white wine

Heat the olive oil and butter together in a heavy skillet over medium-high heat. Add the mushrooms and onion, and sauté until the vegetables start to soften. Add the shrimp, and cook until they're pink all over and the onion is translucent. Stir in the garlic, lemon juice, and wine, and cook for just another minute or two, then serve.

Yield: 3 servings, each with 7 grams of carbohydrates and 1 gram of fiber, for a total of 6 grams of usable carbs and 32 grams of protein.

☉ Smoked Sausage and Sprouts

This is a speeded-up version of a dish in *500 Low-Carb Recipes*—just cut things into smaller bits, and they cook faster!

> 1 pound smoked sausage (500 g)
>
> 2 tablespoons butter
>
> 1 pound brussels sprouts (500 g)
>
> 1/4 cup diced onion (30 g)

Slice the smoked sausage diagonally into 1/2-inch-thick (1-cm-thick) pieces. Melt the butter in a heavy skillet over medium-high heat, and start cooking the sausage in it. Meanwhile, run the Brussels sprouts through the slicing blade of your food processor. Add the Brussels sprouts and onion to the skillet, and continue to cook everything, stirring occasionally until the Brussels sprouts are wilted and the sausage is hot right through. Serve.

Yield: 4 servings, each with 12 grams of carbohydrates and 4 grams of fiber, for a total of 8 grams of usable carbs (less if you choose very low-carb smoked sausage) and 19 grams of protein.

Note: Smoked sausage varies a lot in carb count. Read your labels carefully!

☺ Sour Cream Ham Supper

Another updated, decarbed recipe from Peg Bracken's classic, *The I Hate To Cook Book*.

> 1/2 head cauliflower
>
> 1/2 medium onion, diced
>
> 2 cups cooked ham, cut into strips (200 g)
>
> 8 ounces sliced mushrooms (250 g)
>
> 2 tablespoons butter
>
> 1/2 cup sour cream (100 ml)

Run the cauliflower through the shredding blade of your food processor. Put it in a microwaveable casserole, add a couple of tablespoons of water, cover, and nuke on High for 6 to 7 minutes.

While the cauliflower is cooking, dice the onion and cut the ham into smallish strips. Melt the butter in a large, heavy skillet over medium heat, and sauté the onion, ham, and mushrooms in it, stirring frequently. When the onion is limp and translucent, turn the burner to low and stir in the sour cream. Heat through, but don't let it come to a boil or the sour cream will "crack."

Drain the cauliflower, divide it between 3 plates, and spoon the ham mixture over it.

Yield: 3 servings, each with 9 grams of carbohydrates and 1 gram of fiber, for a total of 8 grams of usable carbs and 19 grams of protein.

☺ Unstuffed Cabbage

Stuffed cabbage is a perennial favorite, but there's no way to stuff all those leaves and get 'em cooked in 15 minutes! Here's a recipe that gives you all the flavor of stuffed cabbage at breakneck speed. Do use very lean ground beef for this recipe—it saves you the time needed to drain off the grease.

> 1 1/2 pounds ground round or other very lean ground beef (750 g)
>
> 1 medium onion, chopped
>
> 1 teaspoon minced garlic or 2 cloves garlic, crushed
>
> 1/2 head cabbage, coarsely chopped
>
> 8-ounce can tomato sauce (250 ml)
>
> 2 tablespoons lemon juice
>
> 1/2 teaspoon pepper
>
> 1/2 teaspoon ground nutmeg
>
> 1/2 teaspoon ground cinnamon
>
> 1 teaspoon salt

Start the ground beef cooking in a heavy skillet over high heat; spread it out to cover the bottom of the pan so it cooks quicker.

While the ground beef is browning, chop the onion and crush the garlic. Plunk them in the pan with the ground beef, and stir it up, using a spatula to turn it over and break it up so that it cooks evenly. Cover the pan and let it continue cooking.

Meanwhile, chop the cabbage coarsely. Stir this into the beef mixture a bit at a time—it will come close to overwhelming your skillet, unless yours is bigger than mine. Again, take care to turn everything over to keep it cooking evenly. Re-cover the pan.

Continue to stir the meat mixture to keep it cooking evenly, covering in between stirrings. When the cabbage is starting to wilt, stir in the tomato sauce, lemon juice, pepper, nutmeg, cinnamon, and salt. Re-cover, let the whole thing simmer for 5 minutes, then serve.

Yield: 5 servings, each with 7 grams of carbohydrates and 2 grams of fiber, for a total of 5 grams of usable carbs and 25 grams of protein.

⏱ Spanish "Rice"

Okay, this isn't really Spanish. It's not even authentically Mexican. And of course it's not rice. But it is passingly like the "Spanish Rice" my mom used to throw together to make a quick, one-dish meal out of hamburger! Feel free to used canned, diced tomatoes without the chilies if you don't like spicy food, although this is really quite mild.

> 1 pound ground round or other very lean ground beef (500 g)
>
> 1 to 2 tablespoons oil
>
> 1/2 head cauliflower
>
> 1/2 green pepper, chopped
>
> 1/2 medium onion, chopped
>
> 1 teaspoon minced garlic
>
> 14.5-ounce can diced tomatoes with green chilies (400 g)
>
> 1/2 teaspoon ground cumin
>
> 1 teaspoon Worcestershire sauce
>
> 1/4 cup water (50 ml)
>
> Salt and pepper

Start browning the beef in the oil over medium-high heat. Meanwhile, run the cauliflower through the shredding blade of your food processor. Put the cauliflower in a microwavable casserole, add a tablespoon or two of water, cover, and microwave on High for just 5 minutes.

Go back to the beef and start breaking it up. When you've got just a little fat in the pan, add the pepper and onion, and sauté them, too. When all the pink is gone from the meat, add the garlic, tomatoes, cumin, Worcestershire sauce, and water, and bring the whole thing to a simmer. Stir in the cauliflower "rice," cover, and let the whole thing simmer for 3 to 5 minutes. Salt and pepper to taste, and serve.

Yield: 4 or 5 servings. Assuming 4 servings, each will have 7 grams of carbohydrates and 1 gram of fiber, for a total of 6 grams of usable carbs and 23 grams of protein.

⊕ Fried "Rice"

This recipe is infinitely variable, and is particularly good for using up any sort of leftover meat you have hanging about. If you don't have any leftovers, feel free to use cooked ham you bought at the grocery store, a can or two of chunk chicken or salad shrimp, or what-have-you.

> 1/2 head cauliflower
>
> Oil
>
> 2 eggs, beaten
>
> 1 1/2 cups diced or shredded leftover cooked meat, canned meat, or seafood (150 g)
>
> 1 cup vegetables* (100 g)
>
> 8 to 10 scallions, sliced, including the crisp part of the green
>
> 2 tablespoons soy sauce
>
> 1/2 teaspoon Splenda

* Use snow peas (chopped into 1-inch [2 cm] pieces), bean sprouts, shredded cabbage, water chestnuts, bamboo shoots—whatever is on hand and sounds good. One or two kinds are better than a mish-mash of half a dozen.

Run the cauliflower through the shredding blade of your food processor. Put the cauliflower in a microwaveable casserole, add a tablespoon or two of water, cover, and microwave on High for 5 minutes.

Spray a medium-size skillet with nonstick cooking spray, and place over medium heat. Add a tablespoon of oil to coat the bottom of the skillet. Pour in the eggs and cover for a minute or so. Let the eggs cook in a flat sheet on the bottom of the skillet. When cooked through, remove and set aside.

Remove the cauliflower from the microwave, and drain it. Put a few tablespoons of oil in a large, heavy skillet or wok, Stir in the meat, vegetables, and scallions. Cook, stirring occasionally, until the veggies are tender-crisp. Add the cauliflower rice, and stir to blend. Shred the sheet of eggs, and stir in the egg strips. Combine the soy sauce with the Splenda, and stir into the fried "rice."

Yield: 2 or 3 servings. Obviously, the carb count on this will vary a little with what ingredients you use. However, assuming that you use the remains of a rotisserie chicken, and half bean sprouts, half snow peas for your vegetables, and that you make 3 servings, each will have 8 grams of carbohydrates and 2 grams of fiber, for a total of 6 grams of usable carbs and 27 grams of protein.

☉ Chicken Chop Suey

    4 tablespoons soy sauce

    2 teaspoons Splenda

    1 1/2 pounds boneless, skinless chicken breast (750 g)

    8 to 10 scallions

    3 to 4 tablespoons oil—peanut or canola is best

    3 cups bean sprouts (150 g)

    3 teaspoons toasted sesame oil

    1/2 teaspoon chicken bouillon granules

    Guar or xanthan

Mix together the soy sauce and Splenda in a little dish, and set aside.

Slice the chicken breast into strips as thin as possible (this is easier to do if it's half-frozen). Cut the scallions into pieces about 1/2 inch (1 cm) long, using all the crisp part of the green.

Assemble all the ingredients by the stove. Place a wok or heavy skillet over highest heat, and add the oil. Give it 30 seconds to 1 minute to heat, then add the chicken. Stir-fry for 4 to 5 minutes, or until the pink is gone. Add the scallions and bean sprouts, and stir-fry for another 1 to 2 minutes. Add the soy sauce mixture, sesame oil, bouillon granules, and a sprinkle of guar or xanthan to thicken the juices. Stir-fry for just another minute, then serve.

Yield: 4 or 5 servings. Assuming 4 servings, each will have 9 grams of carbohydrates and 3 grams of fiber, for a total of 6 grams of usable carbs and 42 grams of protein.

⏲ Hamburger Chop Suey

1 pound ground round or other very lean ground beef (500 g)

2 tablespoons oil

1 medium onion, sliced

2 cups sliced mushrooms (200 g)

2 stalks celery, thinly sliced on the diagonal

1/2 green pepper, diced

1/2 teaspoon minced garlic or 1 clove garlic, crushed

2 cups bean sprouts (100 g)

1/3 cup soy sauce (70 ml)

1/2 teaspoon liquid beef bouillon concentrate

In a wok or large skillet over high heat, start browning the beef in oil and breaking it up. When it's about halfway browned, add the onion, mushrooms, celery, green pepper, and garlic. Continue breaking up the meat while stir-frying the vegetables. When all the pink is gone from the beef and the veggies are almost tender-crisp, add the bean sprouts, soy sauce, and beef bouillon concentrate. Continue stir-frying until the bean sprouts are just barely starting to wilt, then serve.

Yield: 4 servings, each with 8 grams of carbohydrates and 2 grams of fiber, for a total of 6 grams of usable carbs and 24 grams of protein.

⏱ Casual Chan's Special

In my first cookbook, *500 Low-Carb Recipes*, I included a recipe called "Joe," involving hamburger, spinach, and eggs. The original name of that recipe—found in many versions, in many places—was Joe's Special, or Casual Joe's Special. This is a similar recipe with a slight Asian accent, hence the name. This is easy to double, by the way.

> 1/2 pound ground round or other very lean ground beef (250 g)
>
> 1 tablespoon oil
>
> 2 scallions, sliced
>
> 1 cup bean sprouts (50 g)
>
> 2 eggs
>
> 1/2 teaspoon soy sauce
>
> Salt and pepper

Start browning the beef in the oil in a large, heavy skillet over medium-high heat. While it's browning, you can slice the scallions, measure the bean sprouts, and whisk up the eggs together with the soy sauce.

Go back to the stove and start breaking up the beef. When it's crumbled and there's no pink left, add the scallions and sprouts. Stir for a minute or two—just long enough for the veggies to get hot through, but not long enough for the bean sprouts to get limp and soggy. Add the eggs and soy sauce, and scramble until set. Salt and pepper to taste, and serve.

Yield: 2 servings, each with 5 grams of carbohydrates and 1 gram of fiber, for a total of 4 grams of usable carbs and 29 grams of protein.

☺ Beef and Artichoke Skillet

Different and good. Because quite a lot of the carbs in artichokes are in the form of inulin, a very low-impact carb, this is even easier on your blood sugar than the carb count would suggest.

8 slices bacon

1 1/2 pounds boneless beef—sirloin or chuck are fine (750 g)

1/2 medium onion, thinly sliced

2 tablespoons olive oil

1/4 cup cider vinegar (50 ml)

1 tablespoon Splenda

1/2 teaspoon pepper

1/2 teaspoon minced garlic or 1 clove garlic, crushed

14-ounce can quartered artichoke hearts, drained (400 g)

Lay the bacon on a microwave bacon rack or in a glass pie plate. Microwave on High for 8 minutes.

While the bacon is cooking, slice the beef as thinly as you can, then cut across the strips a couple of times, so they're no more than 2 to 3 inches long (5 to 7 cm). (This is easiest if the meat is partly frozen.) Slice up the onion now, too.

Heat the oil in a large, heavy skillet over high heat, and start stir-frying the beef and onion. When the pink is gone from the beef, add the vinegar, Splenda, pepper, garlic, and artichoke hearts, and let the whole thing simmer for 5 minutes or so.

Check on the bacon while the beef is simmering. If it's not crisp yet, give it another minute or so.

Divide the beef mixture between 6 serving plates or bowls, and crumble about a strip and a half of bacon over each portion before serving.

Yield: 6 servings, each with 9 grams of carbohydrates and 4 grams of fiber, for a total of 5 grams of usable carbs and 23 grams of protein.

☉ Sweet and Sour Pork

This is not exactly authentic, because the pork isn't battered and fried. Still, it tastes great! And it's far lower-carb than Sweet and Sour from a Chinese restaurant. If it feels strange to you not to serve this stir-fry over something, there's no reason not to make some cauliflower "rice" to serve with it.

> 3 tablespoons rice or cider vinegar
>
> 1 1/2 tablespoons Splenda
>
> 3 tablespoons canned, crushed pineapple in juice
>
> 1 teaspoon soy sauce
>
> 1/4 teaspoon blackstrap molasses
>
> 1/2 teaspoon minced garlic
>
> 3 tablespoons oil
>
> 12 ounces boneless pork loin, cut into thin strips (375 g)
>
> 1/2 medium green pepper, cut into squares
>
> 1/2 medium onion, sliced
>
> Guar or xanthan

Mix together the vinegar, Splenda, pineapple, soy sauce, molasses, and garlic, and set it by the stove.

Heat the oil in a wok or large skillet over highest heat. Add the pork, and stir-fry until it's half-done. Add the peppers and onions, and keep stir-frying. When all the pink is gone from the pork, add the vinegar mixture, and stir. Let the whole thing simmer for a couple of minutes, stirring once or twice, until the vegetables are tender-crisp. Thicken the pan juices just a touch with guar or xanthan, and serve.

Yield: 2 or 3 servings. Assuming 2 servings, each will have 11 grams of carbohydrates and 1 gram of fiber, for a total of 10 grams of usable carbs and 36 grams of protein.

✻ Each serving also packs 782 milligrams of potassium!

☺ Sweet and Sour Chicken

No big surprise—you can make the same recipe with chicken, instead.

Make the recipe for Sweet and Sour Pork, substituting 12 ounces (375 g) of boneless, skinless chicken breast for the pork.

Yield: 2 or 3 servings. Assuming 2 servings, each will have 11 grams of carbohydrates and 1 gram of fiber, for a total of 10 grams of usable carbs and 39 grams of protein.

✳ The potassium content drops a bit, but you'll still get 479 milligrams.

☺ Mediterranean Turkey Stir Fry

Bright, glorious flavors!

1 1/2 pounds boneless turkey tenderloin, sliced very thinly (750 g)

3 to 4 tablespoons olive oil

1 medium onion, sliced

1 medium green pepper, cut into strips

1/4 cup dry white wine (50 ml)

1/4 cup lemon juice (50 ml)

2.25-ounce can sliced ripe olives, drained (60 g)

2 teaspoons minced garlic or 4 cloves garlic, crushed

1 teaspoon dried oregano

2 teaspoons chicken bouillon crystals

Guar or xanthan

4 tablespoons chopped parsley

In a large skillet or wok, start stir-frying the turkey in the olive oil over high heat. When it's about half-done (half the pink is gone), add the onion and pepper. Continue stir-frying until all the pink is gone from the turkey.

Add the wine, lemon juice, olives, garlic, oregano, and bouillon, and let the whole thing cook, stirring now and then, for another 3 to 4 minutes or until the vegetables are tender-crisp. Thicken the pan juices slightly with the guar or xanthan. Turn off the burner, stir in the parsley, and serve.

Yield: 4 servings, each with 8 grams of carbohydrates and 2 grams of fiber, for a total of 6 grams of usable carbs and 39 grams of protein.

☺ Chicken Asparagus Stir Fry

1 pound asparagus (500 g)

1 medium onion

8 ounces canned sliced water chestnuts, drained (250 g)

¼ cup dry sherry (50 ml)

¼ cup soy sauce (50 ml)

1 teaspoon minced garlic or 2 cloves garlic, crushed

1 ½ pounds boneless, skinless chicken breast, sliced into thin strips (750 g)

¼ cup oil (50 ml)

Guar or xanthan

Snap the ends off the asparagus where they break naturally, and slice diagonally into ½-inch (1-cm) lengths. Slice the onion into thin half-rounds. Open the water chestnuts and drain them. Mix together the sherry, soy sauce, and garlic, and have it sitting by the stove.

Heat the oil in a wok or large skillet over highest heat. Add the chicken and stir-fry for 2 to 3 minutes, or until about half the pink is gone. Add the asparagus and onion, and continue stir-frying until the chicken is cooked through.

Add the water chestnuts and the sherry mixture, stir to combine, and let the whole thing simmer for another 2 to 4 minutes, or until the asparagus is bright green and tender-crisp. Thicken the juices just a little with the guar or xanthan, and serve.

Yield: 4 or 5 servings. Assuming 4 servings, each will have 15 grams of carbohydrates and 3 grams of fiber, for a total of 12 grams of usable carbs and 41 grams of protein.

☉ Ham and Beans Skillet

This is very down-home, which is often a good thing. My husband loves it. You can double this if you like, but your beans will take longer to microwave, possibly taking you a minute or two past the 15-minute mark. Even doubled, though, it's a good, fast supper!

> 6 ounces cooked ham, cut into 1/2-inch (1-cm) cubes (170 g)
>
> 1 tablespoon butter or oil
>
> 2 cups frozen cross-cut green beans (300 g)
>
> 1 tablespoon canned, crushed pineapple in juice
>
> 1 tablespoon low-carbohydrate barbecue sauce
>
> 1/4 teaspoon grated gingerroot
>
> 1/2 teaspoon spicy brown mustard

Start to sauté the ham in the butter or oil over medium heat—you're just browning it a little. While that's happening, put the beans in a microwaveable casserole, add a couple of tablespoons of water, cover, and microwave on High for 7 minutes.

When the microwave goes "ding," check that the beans are done; if they're not, stir them and give them another 2 to 3 minutes. When they're just tender, drain them and add them to the browned ham cubes in the skillet. Add the pineapple, barbecue sauce, gingerroot, and mustard, and stir well. Let it cook for just a minute to blend the flavors, then serve.

Yield: 2 servings, each with 13 grams of carbohydrates and 4 grams of fiber, for a total of 9 grams of usable carbs and 19 grams of protein.

☺ Poultry Hash

This is only a 15-minute recipe if you have leftover turkey or chicken in the house, but you'll be glad to have it that Monday after Thanksgiving, when you've gone back to work and come home to find still more turkey needing to be used up! This tastes good made with the remains of a rotisseried chicken, too.

1/4 head cauliflower

1 medium turnip (a little bigger than a tennis ball)

1/2 medium onion, diced

1 tablespoon butter

2 cups diced leftover turkey or chicken (200 g)

3/4 cup half-and-half (170 ml)

1/2 teaspoon chicken bouillon crystals

1/2 teaspoon poultry seasoning

Guar or xanthan (optional)

Salt and pepper

Whack the cauliflower into a few big chunks and drop it into a food processor with the S-blade in place. Peel the turnip, whack it into quarters, and throw it in there, too. Pulse until everything's chopped to a medium consistency. Dump it into a microwaveable casserole with a lid, add a couple of tablespoons of water, cover it, and nuke it on High for 7 minutes.

Meanwhile, in a big, heavy skillet, start sautéing the onion in the butter over medium heat. While that sautés, dice the leftover fowl.

Add the turkey or chicken to the skillet, and stir it into the onion. By now the cauliflower and turnip should be done; pull them out of the microwave, drain them, and add them to the skillet, too. Stir in the half-and-half, bouillon, and poultry seasoning, cover it, and let it simmer for just a minute or two, to make sure everything is hot all the way through. Thicken it just a tad, if you like, with the guar or xanthan, salt and pepper to taste, and serve.

Yield: 3 servings, each with 8 grams of carbohydrates and 1 gram of fiber, for a total of 7 grams of usable carbs and 24 grams of protein.

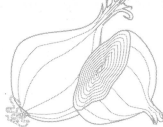

chapter nine

15-Minute Slow Cooker Meals

Okay, I admit it—none of the recipes in this chapter is done in 15 minutes. But that doesn't keep them from being just as convenient—or even more so!—than the recipes in the rest of the book, since they cook happily by themselves while you're out having a life.

With these recipes, the 15-minute limit is on preparation time, not cooking time. All of these recipes require no more than 15 minutes hands-on time, both before cooking and after cooking combined. No spending a half-hour dredging little bits of meat in flour and browning them before you can get your dinner in the slow cooker and your butt out the door, and no coming home from a long day's work to a houseful of hungry people, only to have to add things to your slow cooker meal and then wait an extra half hour. Nope, all these recipes truly are fast and simple—and tasty!

By the way, it's good to know how to speed up or slow down slow cooker food, should you need to: If you want to cut a good hour off your slow cooker recipe, put everything in the crockery liner, put the crockery liner in your microwave oven (this assumes, of course, that your crockery liner lifts out of the electric base, and fits in your microwave—mine does both), and microwave it on 50 percent power for 5 to 10 minutes—just long enough to warm everything through. Then put the crockery liner in the base, cover, and set as per the recipe. To slow a recipe down, you can put the meat in frozen! This will add a good 2 to 3 hours to your cooking time.

⏱ 3-Minute Slow Cooker Pot Roast

This recipe is very 1965, but it's still incredibly easy and it tastes great. Puréed cauliflower "fauxtatoes" are nice with this—they give you something to put the gravy on.

> 8 ounces sliced mushrooms (250 g)
> 2 to 3 pounds boneless chuck pot roast (1 to 1.5 kg)
> 1 envelope French Onion soup mix
> 1/2 cup dry red wine (120 ml)
> Guar or xanthan

Dump the mushrooms in the bottom of your slow cooker and plunk the roast on top of them. Mix together the onion soup mix and wine, and pour it over the whole thing. Slap on the lid, set the slow cooker to Low, and forget about it for 8 hours.

When you come home, fish out the roast (carefully—it will be very tender), and use the guar or xanthan to thicken up the juices in the slow cooker. Serve this gravy with the pot roast.

Yield: Assuming a 2-pound roast (1 kg), this will yield 6 servings. If you eat every drop of the gravy, each serving will have 6 grams of carbohydrates and 1 gram of fiber, for a total of 5 grams of usable carbs and 25 grams of protein.

☉ Pepperoncini Beef

Pepperoncini are hot-but-not-scorching pickled Italian salad peppers —you'll find these in the same aisle as the olives and pickles—and they make this beef very special.

    2 to 3 pounds boneless chuck pot roast (1 to 1.5 kg)

    1 cup pepperoncini peppers, with the vinegar they're packed in (120 g)

    1/2 medium onion, chopped

    Guar or xanthan

    Salt and pepper

Slap the beef in the slow cooker, pour the pepperoncini on top, and strew the onion over that. Put on the lid, set the slow cooker to Low, and leave it for 8 hours.

When it's done, fish out the meat, put it on a platter, and use a slotted spoon to fish out the peppers and pile them on top of the roast. Thicken the juices in the pot with the guar or xanthan, salt and pepper to taste, and serve with the roast.

Yield: Assuming a 2-pound roast (1 kg), this will yield 6 servings, each with 3 grams of carbohydrates, a trace of fiber, and 24 grams of protein.

⏱ Caribbean Slow Cooker Lamb

I buy whole legs of lamb and have the butcher at the grocery store cut them up for me—a smallish roast from each end, and steaks from the middle. They never charge for this service, and this gives me lamb roasts small enough to fit in my slow cooker. The problem ingredient here is the tamarind concentrate—look in a grocery store with a good International section. I found it in a medium-size town in southern Indiana, so you may well find it near you! If you can't find it, you could use a tablespoon of lemon juice and a teaspoon of Splenda, instead, and your lamb will be less authentically Caribbean-tasting, but still yummy.

2- to 3-pound section of a leg of lamb (1 to 1.5 kg)

1/2 medium onion, chopped

1/2 teaspoon minced garlic or 1 clove garlic, crushed

1 teaspoon tamarind concentrate

1 tablespoon spicy brown mustard

1 cup canned diced tomatoes (250 ml)

1 teaspoon hot sauce—preferably Caribbean Scotch Bonnet
   sauce—or more or less, to taste

Guar or xanthan

Salt and pepper

Place the lamb in the slow cooker. Stir together the onion, garlic, tamarind, mustard, tomatoes, and hot sauce, and pour over the lamb. Set the cooker on Low, and let it cook for a good 8 hours.

When it's done, remove the lamb to a serving platter, thicken the pot juices with the guar or xanthan if it seems necessary, salt and pepper to taste, and serve.

Yield: Assuming a 2 1/2-pound (1.2 kg) section of a leg of lamb, this will be 6 servings, each with 5 grams of carbohydrates and a trace of fiber (if you eat all the gravy—fewer carbs if you don't), and 27 grams of protein.

◷ Slow Cooker Chicken Guadeloupe

This isn't authentically anything, but it borrows its flavors from the Creole cooking of the Caribbean.

1 cut-up broiler-fryer chicken, about 3 1/2 pounds (1.5 to 2 kg), or whatever chicken parts you prefer (1.5 to 2 kg)

1/2 medium onion, chopped

2 teaspoons ground allspice

1 teaspoon dried thyme

1/4 cup lemon juice; bottled is fine (50 ml)

1 can (400 g canned) diced tomatoes with chilies

1 shot (3 tablespoons) dark rum

Guar or xanthan

Salt and pepper

Just throw the chicken, onion, allspice, thyme, lemon juice, chilies, and rum in the slow cooker, set it to Low, and let it go for 5 to 6 hours. Fish out the chicken carefully—it'll be sliding from the bone! Thicken up the stuff in the pot with the guar or xanthan, salt and pepper to taste, and serve over the chicken.

Yield: 5 or 6 servings. Assuming 5 servings, each will have 6 grams of carbohydrates and 1 gram of fiber, for a total of 5 grams of usable carbs and 35 grams of protein.

☺ Sort of Ethiopian Chicken Stew

Again, the slow cooker method is hardly authentic, but the flavors come from an Ethiopian recipe—except that the Ethiopians would use a lot more cayenne! Increase it if you like really hot food.

> 1 cut-up broiler-fryer, about 3 pounds (1.5 kg)
>
> 1 medium onion, chopped
>
> 1 teaspoon cayenne
>
> 1 teaspoon paprika
>
> 1/2 teaspoon pepper
>
> 1/2 teaspoon grated gingerroot
>
> 2 tablespoons lemon juice
>
> 1/2 cup water (120 ml)
>
> Guar or xanthan
>
> Salt and pepper

Throw the chicken, onion, cayenne, paprika, pepper, gingerroot, lemon juice, and water in your slow cooker, and set it to Low. Leave it for 5 to 6 hours. If you'd like to make this really stewlike, you can pick the meat off the bones when it's done (which will be very easy), thicken the gravy with guar or xanthan, and then stir the chicken back into the liquid. Or you can just serve the gravy over the chicken. Take your pick.

Yield: 5 or 6 servings. Assuming 5 servings, each will have 3 grams of carbohydrates and 1 gram of fiber, for a total of 2 grams of usable carbs and 35 grams of protein.

⊕ Chipotle Turkey Legs

Spicy, rich Southwestern flavor.

3 turkey legs

1 1/2 teaspoons cumin

1 teaspoon chili powder

1 teaspoon dried, powdered sage

1 teaspoon minced garlic or 2 cloves garlic, crushed

1/2 teaspoon red pepper flakes

1/4 teaspoon turmeric

1 or 2 canned chipotle chilies in adobo sauce, plus a couple
   of teaspoons of the sauce they come in

8 ounces tomato sauce (250 ml)

1 tablespoon Worcestershire sauce

6 tablespoons shredded queso quesadilla (optional)*

Guar or xanthan

* This is a mild, white Mexican cheese. Monterey Jack is an acceptable substitute.

Plunk the turkey legs in the slow cooker. (If you can fit more, feel free. My slow cooker will only hold 3.) Put the cumin, chili powder, sage, garlic, red pepper flakes, turmeric, chilies, tomato sauce, and Worcestershire sauce in the blender, run it for a minute, then pour the mixture over the turkey legs. Cover, turn the slow cooker to Low, and leave it for 5 to 6 hours.

When it's done, remove each turkey leg to a serving plate, thicken the juices in the pot with guar or xanthan, and spoon over the turkey legs. If you like, sprinkle 2 tablespoons of shredded cheese over each turkey leg and let it melt for a minute or two before serving.

Yield: 3 servings, each with 8 grams of carbohydrates and 2 grams of fiber, for a total of 6 grams of usable carbs and—depending on the size of the turkey legs—40 to 50 grams of protein.

Note: Chipotle peppers are smoked jalapeños. They're very different from regular jalapeños, and they're quite delicious. Look for them, canned in adobo sauce, in the Mexican foods section of big grocery stores. Since you're unlikely to use the whole can at once, you'll be happy to know that you can store your chipotles in the freezer, where they'll live happily for months and stay pliable enough that you can peel one off when you want to use it.

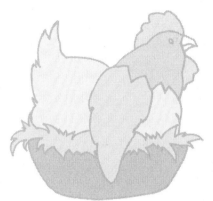

◔ Choucroute Garni

This is a streamlined version of a traditional dish from the Alsace region of France—the name means Garnished Sauerkraut. So simple and so good, especially on a cold night.

14-ounce can red sauerkraut (400 g)

1 tablespoon bacon grease

1/4 cup apple cider vinegar (50 ml)

1 tablespoon Splenda

1/2 medium onion, thinly sliced

2 tablespoons gin

1/4 cup dry white wine (50 ml)

1 pound meat—your choice of any combination of kielbasa,
   smoked sausage, frankfurters, link sausages, 1/4-inch-thick (5 mm)
   ham slices, smoked pork chops* (500 g)

* I use 1/2 pound (250 g) each of the lowest carbohydrate kielbasa and smoked sausage I can find.

Dump your sauerkraut into a colander, rinse lightly, drain, and dump into the slow cooker. Add the bacon grease, vinegar, Splenda, onion, gin, and wine, and give it a quick stir. Plunk the meat on top, cover the slow cooker, and set it to Low. Cook for 5 to 6 hours.

Yield: 3 or 4 servings. Assuming 3 servings and depending on what meats you use, each will have in the neighborhood of 9 grams of carbohydrates and 3 grams of fiber, for a total of 6 grams of usable carbs (you can cut this by using the very lowest carbohydrate sausages you can find) and roughly 16 grams of protein.

Note: This doesn't even start to fill my slow cooker, so feel free to double or even triple this recipe. If you increase it, I'd layer it—a layer of kraut, a layer of meat, a layer of kraut, and so on. And, of course, you'll have to increase the cooking time by an hour, maybe two, depending on how many extra layers you use.

Slow Cooker Ribs

We just love ribs around here, but I've never thought of them as something "quick and easy." Then I thought of putting them in the slow cooker. Wow!

Slow cooker ribs aren't exactly like ribs done over a slow fire, of course, but they're incredibly tasty and falling-off-the-bone tender. What's more, they're really, really easy. Here are a few ideas on how to cook ribs in a slow cooker.

☺ Rosemary-Ginger Ribs with Apricot Glaze

Blue Slaw—or any coleslaw—is good with these. Also, feel free to use a full-size slab of ribs—about 6 pounds (3 kg) worth—and double the seasonings if you're feeding a family.

> 1 slab baby back ribs, about 2 1/2 pounds (about 1 kg)
>
> Purchased Rosemary-Ginger Rub (Stubb's makes this)
>
> 2 tablespoons low-sugar apricot preserves
>
> 1 1/2 teaspoons spicy brown mustard
>
> 1 teaspoon Splenda
>
> 1 1/2 teaspoons soy sauce

Sprinkle both sides of the slab of ribs generously with the Rosemary-Ginger Rub. Curl the slab of ribs around and fit it down into your slow cooker. Cover, and set the slow cooker on Low. Forget about it for 9 to 10 hours. (No, I didn't forget anything. You don't put any liquid in the slow cooker. Don't sweat it.)

When the time's up, mix together the preserves, mustard, Splenda, and soy sauce. Carefully remove the ribs from the slow cooker—they may fall apart on you a bit, they'll be so tender. Arrange them meaty-side-up on a broiler rack. Spread the apricot glaze evenly over the ribs and run them under a broiler set on High, 3 to 4 inches (7 to 10 cm) from the heat, for 7 to 8 minutes, then serve.

Yield: 2 or 3 servings. Assuming 3 servings, each will have 5 grams of carbohydrates, a trace of fiber, and 38 grams of protein.

☉ Slow Cooker "Barbecued" Ribs

Okay, it's not really barbecue, because it's not done over a fire. But this recipe tastes great and lets you dig into your ribs within minutes of walking in the door.

> 1 slab baby back ribs, about 2 1/2 pounds (about 1 kg)
>
> Memphis-Style Dry Rub (page 222, or you can purchase good
>   dry rub in most grocery stores)
>
> 1/4 cup Reduced-Carb Spicy Barbecue Sauce (see page 226)
>   or 1/4 cup purchased low-carb barbecue sauce* (50 ml)

* Atkins makes one, and so does Walden—these are both available through online retailers. There's also a brand called Stubb's, pretty widely distributed in grocery stores, that has less than half the sugar of most commercial barbecue sauces and tastes great. That's what I use.

Sprinkle the slab of ribs liberally on both sides with the dry rub, coil the ribs up, and slide them into your slow cooker. Cover, set to Low, and let them go for 9 to 10 hours.

When dinnertime rolls around, pull the ribs out of the slow cooker—as in the previous recipe, do this carefully because they'll be falling-apart tender.
Lay the ribs on a broiler rack, meaty side up, and spread the barbecue sauce over them. Broil 3 to 4 inches (7 to 10 cm) from the broiler set on High for 7 to 8 minutes, then serve.

Yield: Your carb count will be a bit different depending on whether you use homemade sugar-free barbecue sauce or commercial low-carb sauce. If 3 people share these, each will get about 5 grams of carbohydrates, no fiber, and 38 grams of protein.

> **Note:** If you'd like to give these a smoked flavor, you can buy liquid smoke flavoring at your grocery store. Simply brush the ribs with the liquid smoke before you sprinkle on the dry rub.

⏱ Slow Cooker Teriyaki Ribs

Sweet, spicy, and tangy, and falling-off-the-bone tender. The 15-minute time frame does not include making the ketchup, but the teriyaki sauce should fit in, and you'll want to have ketchup on hand all the time, anyway.

6 pounds pork spare ribs, cut into 3 or 4 pieces so they fit in the pot (about 3 kg)

3/4 cup Dana's No-Sugar Ketchup or commercial no-sugar ketchup (170 ml)

1 batch Teriyaki Sauce (see page 228)

1/4 cup Splenda (30 g)

1/4 teaspoon blackstrap molasses

1 teaspoon minced garlic or 2 cloves garlic, crushed

Guar or xanthan

Plop the ribs in the slow cooker. Mix the ketchup, teriyaki sauce, Splenda, molasses, and garlic together, pour it into the cooker, cover the pot, and set it on Low. Forget it for 10 hours.

When the time's up, use tongs to pull out the now unbelievably tender and flavorful ribs. Ladle out as much of the pot liquid as you think you'll use, and thicken it using the guar or xanthan. Serve the sauce over the ribs.

Yield: 6 servings, each with roughly 3 grams of carbohydrates, a trace of fiber (depending on how much of the liquid you eat), and 48 grams of protein.

☺ "I've Got a Life" Chicken

This is remarkably good—sweet and tangy and fruity. It takes just about the whole 15 minutes—about 12 to get it into the pot, and another couple at the far end for thickening the sauce—but it's worth it.

> 3 to 3 ½ pounds (1.5 to 2 kg) bone-in chicken parts of your choice—I use legs and thighs, but a whole cut up chicken would work great (1.5 to 2 kg)
>
> 8 ounces sliced mushrooms (250 g)
>
> 3 tablespoons orange juice
>
> Grated zest of one orange
>
> 1 tablespoon chicken bouillon crystals
>
> ½ teaspoon pepper
>
> 8-ounce can tomato sauce (250 ml)
>
> 2 tablespoons soy sauce
>
> 2 tablespoons Splenda
>
> ½ teaspoon blackstrap molasses
>
> 2 teaspoons minced garlic or 4 cloves garlic, crushed
>
> 1 teaspoon dried thyme
>
> Guar or xanthan

Remove the skin and any big lumps of fat from the chicken, and throw it in the slow cooker. (You can save time by buying chicken with the skin already removed, but it's more expensive.) Dump the mushrooms on top.

Mix together the orange juice, orange zest, bouillon, pepper, tomato sauce, soy sauce, Splenda, molasses, garlic, and thyme, and dump it on top of the chicken and mushrooms. Cover the pot, set it to Low, and let it cook for 5 to 6 hours.

When it's done, pull the chicken out and put it on a platter. Use the guar or xanthan to thicken up the sauce in the pot, and serve it with the chicken.

Yield: 5 or 6 servings. Assuming 6 servings, each will have 8 grams of carbohydrates and 1 gram of fiber, for a total of 7 grams of usable carbs (assuming you eat all of the gravy) and 31 grams of protein.

⊕ Slow Cooker Brewery Chicken and Vegetables

Plenty of vegetables in here, so you don't need a thing with it, except maybe some bread for the carb-eaters in the family. And the gravy comes out a beautiful color!

8 ounces turnips (two turnips roughly the size of tennis balls),
    peeled and cut in chunks (250 g)

2 stalks celery, sliced

1 medium carrot, scrubbed and sliced

1/2 medium onion, sliced

1 tablespoon chicken bouillon granules

2 1/2 to 3 pounds cut-up chicken—I use leg and thigh quarters,
    cut apart at the joint. (1 to 1.5 kg)

1 can very low-carb light beer—Miller Lite, Milwaukee's Best Light,
    or Michelob Ultra

14.5-ounce can diced tomatoes with green chilies (400 g)

Guar or xanthan (optional)

Salt and pepper

Just put the turnips, celery, carrot, onion, bouillon, and chicken in the slow cooker in the order given. Pour the beer and the tomatoes over the lot, cover it, and set the slow cooker to Low. Cook for 8 to 9 hours.

When it's done, use tongs to pull out the chicken, and place it on a serving platter. Then, using a slotted spoon, scoop out the vegetables. Put 1 1/2 cups (350 ml) of them in the blender, and pile the rest on and around the chicken on the platter. Scoop out 1 1/2 to 2 cups (350 to 500 ml) of the liquid left in the slow cooker and put it in the blender with the vegetables. Purée the veggies and broth, and thicken the mixture a little more with the guar or xanthan, if it seems necessary. Salt and pepper to taste, and serve as a sauce with the chicken and vegetables.

Yield: 5 or 6 servings. Assuming 5 servings, each will have 8 grams of carbohydrates and 2 grams of fiber, for a total of 6 grams of usable carbs and 36 grams of protein.

☉ Chicken Chili Verde

This is marvelous, and a really nice change from the traditional beef chili.

1 1/2 pounds boneless, skinless chicken breasts (750 g)

1 1/2 cups bottled salsa verde (350 ml)

1/2 medium onion, chopped

1 bay leaf

1/2 teaspoon pepper

1 teaspoon ground cumin

1 teaspoon minced garlic or 2 cloves garlic, crushed

1 to 2 tablespoons jarred, sliced jalapeños*

2 teaspoons chicken bouillon granules

Guar or xanthan (optional)

Sour cream

Shredded Monterey Jack cheese

Chopped fresh cilantro

* I used 2 tablespoons, and it came out fairly hot.

Just plunk the chicken breasts into your slow cooker, and throw the salsa verde, onion, bay leaf, pepper, cumin, garlic, jalapeños, and bouillon on top. Cover it, set it to Low, and let it cook for 9 to 10 hours.

When the time's up, take a fork and shred the chicken right there in the pot, which will now be very easy to do. Stir it up, thicken the chili a little with the guar or xanthan if you think it needs it, and serve with sour cream, shredded cheese, and chopped cilantro on top.

Yield: 5 servings, each with 7 grams of carbohydrates, a trace of fiber, and 31 grams of protein (before adding garnishes).

Note: Leftover Chicken Chili Verde makes great omelets, especially combined with Monterey Jack cheese!

chapter ten

15-Minute Side Dishes

I think these side dishes make very nice accompaniments to simple protein dishes—a grilled or pan-broiled steak or chop, a rotisserie chicken from the grocery store, or something like that. Of course, if you do both a 15-minute side dish *and* a 15-minute main course, you're looking at a bit more than 15 minutes total cooking time (although not necessarily 30 minutes, since you may well be able to multi-task).

When you *don't* feel like taking the time and effort to make one of these side dishes, or when your entire 15 minutes is going into making your main course, the easiest sides are frozen vegetables or bagged salad with bottled dressing. Nothing wrong with either of these, and we'll talk a little about them at the end of the chapter.

We start this section with a couple of basic recipes that every low-carber needs. These are taken from my previous book, *500 Low-Carb Recipes*: Fauxtatoes, a cauliflower purée that makes a great substitute for mashed potatoes, and Cauliflower "Rice," cauliflower run through the shredding blade of a food processor. These two recipes are repeated because they're great for serving with any dish that has a sauce or gravy. Either one of these is the obvious side, for instance, with any of the slow cooker dishes that makes a lot of good, flavorful gravy.

After these two recipes, you'll find a variety of ways to season Cauliflower Rice—I've become quite enchanted with this wonderful food, as you'll see! All these recipes start the same way—you run a half a head of cauliflower through a food processor's shredding blade, and microwave it. If, like me, you discover that you're very fond of this wonderfully versatile food, you might consider running a couple of heads of cauliflower through the food processor over the weekend and storing the resultant cauliflower "rice" in a large zipper-lock bag in the refrigerator, to draw on through the week. However, all of these recipes fit into the 15-minute limit, including the minute or two needed to shred the cauliflower.

There are also recipes here where the cauliflower is sliced or chunked. Indeed, there are more recipes for cauliflower than any other vegetable here, because cauliflower is The Great Fooler and makes a terrific substitute for rice, potatoes, and even bulgar wheat or noodles. And, of course, cauliflower is more nutritious than any of these!

By the way, don't bother cutting the core out of the cauliflower—just trim off the leaves and the very base of the stem, whack the whole thing into chunks, and shred up the core and stem along with the flowerets. If you core the cauliflower, it will still work fine, but the yield for these recipes will be somewhat less.

☺ Cauliflower Puree, a.k.a. Fauxtatoes

This is a wonderful substitute for mashed potatoes with any dish that has a gravy or sauce. Feel free, by the way, to use frozen cauliflower instead; it works quite well here.

> 1 head cauliflower or 1 1/2 pounds frozen cauliflower (750 g)
>
> 4 tablespoons butter
>
> Salt and pepper

Put the cauliflower in a microwaveable casserole with a lid, add a couple of tablespoons of water, and cover. Nuke it on High for 10 to 12 minutes, or until quite tender but not sulfury smelling. (You may steam or boil the cauliflower, if you prefer.) Drain it thoroughly, and put it through the blender or food processor until it's well puréed. Add butter, salt, and pepper to taste.

Yield: At least 6 generous servings, each with 5 grams of carbohydrates and 2 grams of fiber, for a total of 3 grams of usable carbs and 2 grams of protein.

☉ Cauliflower Rice

With thanks to Fran McCullough! I got this idea from her book *Living Low Carb*, and it's served me very well, indeed.

> ¹/₂ head cauliflower
> Butter (optional)

Simply put the cauliflower through your food processor using the shredding blade. This gives a texture that is remarkably similar to rice. You can steam this, microwave it, or even sauté it in butter. I virtually always microwave it, usually for 7 minutes on High, as you'll see in all the following recipes. Whatever you do, though, don't overcook it!

Yield: This is at least 3 or 4 servings. Assuming 3 servings, each will have 5 grams of carbohydrates and 2 grams of fiber, for a total of 3 grams of usable carbs and 2 grams of protein.

☺ Blue Cheese-Scallion "Risotto"

Since West Coasters call scallions "green onions," I toyed with calling this
"Blue-Green 'Risotto'." Making risotto out of cauliflower "rice" is one of the
best ideas I've ever had!

1/2 head cauliflower

8 scallions, thinly sliced

2/3 cup diced green pepper (80 g)

1 tablespoon butter

1 tablespoon olive oil

1 teaspoon chicken bouillon granules

1/4 cup dry white wine (50 ml)

1/4 cup crumbled blue cheese (30 g)

1/4 cup grated Parmesan cheese (30 g)

2 tablespoons heavy cream

Put the cauliflower through the food processor using the shredding blade.
Put it in a microwaveable casserole, add a couple of tablespoons of water, cover,
and microwave on High for 7 minutes.

While that's nuking, slice the scallions and dice the pepper. Then, in a large,
heavy skillet over medium heat, start sautéing the scallions and pepper in
the butter and oil.

When the microwave goes "ding," remove the cauliflower and drain it. When the
green pepper is starting to get soft, add the cauliflower to the skillet and stir it in.
Then stir in the bouillon, white wine, blue cheese, Parmesan cheese, and heavy
cream. Cook for another 3 to 4 minutes, and serve.

Yield: 5 servings, each with 4 grams of carbohydrates and 1 gram of fiber, for a total
of 3 grams of usable carbs and 4 grams of protein.

⊕ Mushroom "Risotto"

Man, is this good! One of the best side dishes I've ever come up with.

> 1/2 head cauliflower
>
> 3 tablespoons butter
>
> 1 cup sliced mushrooms (100 g)
>
> 1/2 medium onion, diced
>
> 1 teaspoon minced garlic or 2 cloves garlic
>
> 2 tablespoons dry vermouth
>
> 1 tablespoon chicken bouillon granules
>
> 3/4 cup grated Parmesan cheese (100 g)
>
> Guar or xanthan
>
> 2 tablespoons chopped fresh parsley (60 ml)

Run the cauliflower through the food processor using the shredding blade. Put the cauliflower in a microwaveable casserole, add a couple of tablespoons of water, cover, and microwave on High for 7 minutes.

While the cauliflower is nuking, melt the butter over medium-high heat and add the mushrooms, onion, and garlic, and sauté them all together.

When the cauliflower is done, pull it out of the microwave and drain it. When the mushrooms have changed color and are looking done, add the cauliflower and stir everything together. Stir in the vermouth, bouillon, and cheese, and let the whole thing cook for another 2 to 3 minutes. Sprinkle just a little guar or xanthan over the "risotto," stirring all the while, to give it a creamy texture. Stir in the parsley, and serve.

Yield: 5 servings, each with 4 grams of carbohydrates and 1 gram of fiber, for a total of 3 grams of usable carbs and 6 grams of protein.

☺ Saffron "Rice"

What a brilliant color! This looks so beautiful on your plate. Good with any main dish that's a little fruity-spicy.

- 1/2 head cauliflower
- 1 teaspoon saffron threads
- 1/4 cup water (50 ml)
- 1/2 medium onion, chopped
- 1 teaspoon minced garlic or 2 cloves garlic, crushed
- 2 tablespoons butter
- 2 teaspoons chicken bouillon granules
- 1/4 cup chopped toasted almonds (30 g)

Run the cauliflower through the food processor using the shredding blade. Put the cauliflower in a microwaveable casserole, add a couple of tablespoons of water, cover, and microwave on High for 7 minutes.

Start soaking the saffron threads in the water. While that's happening, sauté the onion and garlic in the butter over medium heat in a large, heavy skillet.

When the cauliflower is done, remove it from the microwave, drain it, and add it to the skillet. Pour in the water and saffron, and stir in the chicken bouillon granules. Let the whole thing cook together for a minute or two while you chop the almonds. Stir the almonds into the "rice" and serve.

Yield: 5 servings of brilliantly yellow "rice," each with 4 grams of carbohydrates and 1 gram of fiber, for a total of 3 grams of usable carbs and 2 grams of protein.

Variation: Traditionally, saffron rice has raisins in it. If you can afford the extra carbohydrates—if, for instance, you're serving a very low-carb main dish—you can stir in 3 tablespoons of raisins with the saffron and water. Each serving of this version will have 8 grams of carbohydrates and 1 gram of fiber, for a total of 7 grams of usable carbs and 2 grams of protein.

Note: Saffron is the most expensive spice in the world, and with good reason. Each saffron thread is the stamen of a particular kind of crocus flower. There are four per flower, and they all have to be plucked by hand, with tweezers. It takes 50,000 of them to make a pound (500 g) of saffron! Luckily, small quantities of saffron make a big impact on a dish. Do look for saffron in a store that sells bulk spices—many health food stores do. At least that way you're not paying extra for that little glass jar.

☺ Chicken-Almond "Rice"

This is great for all of you who miss Rice-a-Roni and similar products. And it's terrific with a simple rotisseried chicken.

> ¹/₂ head cauliflower
>
> ¹/₂ medium onion, chopped
>
> 2 tablespoons butter
>
> 1 tablespoon chicken bouillon granules
>
> 1 teaspoon poultry seasoning
>
> ¹/₄ cup dry white wine (50 ml)
>
> ¹/₄ cup sliced or slivered almonds (30 g)

Run the cauliflower through the food processor using the shredding blade. Put the cauliflower in a microwaveable casserole, add a couple of tablespoons of water, cover, and microwave on High for 7 minutes.

While that's cooking, sauté the onion in 1 tablespoon of butter in a large, heavy skillet over medium-high heat.

When the cauliflower is done, pull it out of the microwave, drain it, and add it to the skillet. Add the chicken bouillon granules, poultry seasoning, and wine, and stir. Turn the burner down to low heat.

Let that simmer for a minute or two while you sauté the almonds in the remaining tablespoon of butter in a small, heavy skillet. When the almonds are golden, stir them into the "rice," and serve.

Yield: 5 servings, each with 4 grams of carbohydrates and 1 gram of fiber, for a total of 3 grams of usable carbs and 2 grams of protein.

> **Note:** Sunkist now puts out sliced, toasted almonds in various flavors, under the name "Almond Accents." Feel free to use these to vary this dish!

☺ Beef and Bacon "Rice" with Pine Nuts

1/2 head cauliflower

4 strips bacon

1/2 medium onion, chopped

1 tablespoon liquid beef bouillon concentrate

2 tablespoons tomato sauce

2 tablespoons toasted pine nuts

2 tablespoons chopped parsley

Run the cauliflower through the food processor using the shredding blade, put it in a microwaveable casserole, add a couple of tablespoons of water, cover it, and nuke it on High for 7 minutes.

While that's cooking, cut the bacon into little pieces—kitchen shears are good for this—and start the little bacon bits frying in a heavy skillet over medium-high heat. When a little grease has cooked out of the bacon, throw the onion into the skillet. Fry them until the onion is translucent and the bacon is browned and getting crisp.

By now the cauliflower should be done. Drain it and throw it in the skillet with the bacon and onion. Add the beef bouillon concentrate and tomato sauce, and stir the whole thing up to combine everything—you can add a couple of tablespoons of water, if you like, to help the liquid flavorings spread.

Stir in the pine nuts and parsley (you can just snip it right into the skillet with those kitchen shears), and serve.

Yield: 4 or 5 servings. Assuming 4 servings, each will have 3 grams of carbohydrates and 1 gram of fiber, for a total of 2 grams of usable carbs and 4 grams of protein.

☺ Not-Quite-Middle-Eastern Salad

Here shredded cauliflower stands in for bulgar wheat instead of rice. This salad is incredibly delicious, incredibly nutritious, and quite beautiful on the plate. Plus it gets better after a couple of days in the fridge, so taking an extra few minutes to double the batch is definitely worth it.

1/2 head cauliflower

2/3 cup sliced stuffed olives (70 g)*

7 scallions, sliced

2 cups triple-washed fresh spinach, finely chopped (50 g)

1 stalk celery, diced

1 small ripe tomato, finely diced

4 tablespoons chopped parsley

1/4 cup olive oil (50 ml)

1 teaspoon minced garlic or 2 cloves garlic, crushed

1 tablespoon red wine vinegar

2 tablespoons mayonnaise

Salt and pepper

*You can buy sliced stuffed olives in jars.

Run the cauliflower through the food processor using the shredding blade, put it in a microwaveable casserole, add a couple of tablespoons of water, cover the dish, and nuke it on High for just 5 minutes.

While that's cooking, put the olives, scallions, spinach, celery, tomato, and parsley in a large salad bowl.

When the cauliflower comes out of the microwave, dump it in a strainer and run cold water over it for a moment or two to cool it. (If you don't care about your salad being ready to eat in 15 minutes' time, you can let the cauliflower cool, uncovered, instead.) Drain the cauliflower well, and dump it in with all the other vegetables. Add the oil, garlic, vinegar, and mayonnaise, and toss. Salt and pepper to taste, toss again, and serve.

Yield: 6 servings, each with 5 grams of carbohydrates and 2 grams of fiber, for a total of 3 grams of usable carbs and 1 gram of protein.

☾ Cauliflower Parmesan

Wonderful with a simple broiled or grilled steak, and easy to make while that steak is cooking.

> ¹/₂ head cauliflower
>
> ¹/₂ cup heavy cream (120 ml)
>
> ¹/₂ cup grated Parmesan cheese (50 g)
>
> Salt and pepper

Run the cauliflower through the slicing disk on your food processor. Put it in a microwaveble casserole, add a couple of tablespoons of water, cover, and microwave on High for 4 minutes. When the cauliflower comes out of the microwave, drain it and put it in a large, heavy skillet you've sprayed with nonstick cooking spray. Reduce the heat to low. Add the cream and Parmesan, stir, cover, and let the whole thing simmer for 5 minutes or so. Salt and pepper to taste, then serve.

Yield: 4 servings, each with 2 grams of carbohydrates, a trace of fiber, and 5 grams of protein.

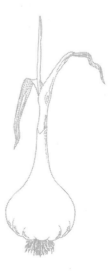

◷ Little Mama's Side Dish

Just the thing with a simple dinner of broiled chops or a steak, and it's even good all by itself. Beautiful to look at, too, what with all those colors.

> 4 slices bacon
>
> 1/2 head cauliflower
>
> 1/2 green pepper
>
> 1/2 medium onion
>
> 1/4 cup sliced stuffed olives (30 g)*

*You can buy sliced stuffed olives in jars.

Chop the bacon into small bits and start it frying in a large, heavy skillet over medium-high heat. (Give the skillet a squirt of nonstick cooking spray first.)

Chop the cauliflower into bits about 1/2 inch (1 cm) chunks. Chop up the stem, too; no need to waste it. Put the chopped cauliflower in a microwaveable casserole with a lid, add a couple of tablespoons of water, cover, and microwave for 7 minutes on High.

Give the bacon a stir, then it's back to the chopping board. Dice the pepper and onion. By now some fat has cooked out of the bacon and it is starting to brown around the edges. Add the pepper and onion to the skillet. Sauté until the onion is translucent and the pepper is starting to get soft.

By the time that confluence of events transpires, the cauliflower should be done. Add it to the skillet without draining, and stir—the extra little bit of water is going to help to dissolve the yummy bacon flavor from the bottom of the skillet and carry it through the dish.

Stir in the olives, let the whole thing cook another minute while stirring, then serve.

Yield: 4 or 5 servings. Assuming 5 servings, each will have 3 grams of carbohydrates and 1 gram of fiber, for a total of 2 grams of usable carbs and 2 grams of protein.

☉ Easy Garlic Creamed Spinach

This is about the easiest creamed spinach ever, and quite good too.

> Two 10-ounce boxes frozen chopped spinach, thawed (600 g)
>   or two 10-ounce bags triple-washed fresh spinach (600 g)
> 1 tablespoon butter
> 5.2-ounce package creamy garlic-herb cheese, like Boursin or Alouette (150 g)

If you're using fresh spinach, you might coarsely chop it, quickly. Melt the butter in a large, heavy skillet, and add the spinach. Cook, stirring, for 3 to 4 minutes—you want fresh spinach just barely wilted and frozen spinach just well-heated through.

Cut the cheese into a few chunks and add it to the skillet. Stir until the cheese is completely melted, then serve.

Yield: 6 servings, each with 4 grams of carbohydrates and 3 grams of fiber, for a total of 1 gram of usable carbs and 4 grams of protein.

☺ Sour Cream Spinach

My husband liked this so much, he yummed down the whole batch.

> 10-ounce package frozen chopped spinach (300 g)
>
> 1/4 medium onion
>
> 2 tablespoons butter
>
> 1/3 cup sour cream (70 ml)
>
> 1 teaspoon cider vinegar

Unwrap the spinach and put it in a microwaveable casserole with a lid. Add a couple of tablespoons of water, cover, and zap it on High for 5 minutes.

Meanwhile, in a large, heavy skillet, start sautéing the onion in the butter over medium-high heat.

When the microwave goes "ding," check to see if the spinach is done—you want it good and hot right through, but not cooked to death. If there's still a cold spot in the middle, stir it and put it back for another 2 minutes on High.

When the spinach is cooked and the onion is translucent, drain the spinach and stir it into the onion, combining well. Stir in the sour cream and the vinegar, heat it through without letting it simmer, then serve.

Yield: 3 servings, each with 6 grams of carbohydrates and 3 grams of fiber, for a total of 3 grams of usable carbs and 4 grams of protein.

⊕ Lemon-Mustard Asparagus

A simple variation of the traditional Asparagus with Lemon Butter in *500 Low-Carb Recipes*.

> 1 pound asparagus (500 g)
> 3 tablespoons butter
> 1 1/2 teaspoons lemon juice
> 1 1/2 teaspoons spicy brown or Dijon mustard

Snap the ends off the asparagus spears where they break naturally. Put the asparagus in a microwaveable casserole, or lay it flat in a glass pie plate. Add a couple of tablespoons of water, cover (use plastic wrap or a plate to cover a pie plate), and microwave on High for 3 to 4 minutes.

While the asparagus is cooking, melt the butter over low heat, and stir in the lemon juice and mustard. (If you prefer, you can wait until the asparagus is cooked and melt the butter in the microwave, too.)

When the asparagus comes out of the microwave, uncover it right away or it will continue to cook and become gray and mushy within 5 minutes! Arrange on 4 serving plates, and divide the lemon-mustard sauce between the servings.

Yield: 4 servings, each with 3 grams of carbohydrates and 1 gram of fiber, for a total of 2 grams of usable carbs and 2 grams of protein.

☉ Aparagus Parmesan

If you're paying really close attention, you'll notice that this is the asparagus from the Asparagi All'uovo (see page 47), without the eggs. It's a great side dish with a simple chicken breast.

> 1 pound asparagus (500 g)
>
> 1/2 teaspoon minced garlic or 1 clove garlic, crushed
>
> 1/4 cup olive oil (50 ml)
>
> Salt and pepper
>
> 1/2 cup grated Parmesan cheese* (50 g)

* Using good-quality cheese instead of the cheap stuff in the green shaker pays off here.

Snap the bottoms off the asparagus spears where they break naturally. Put the asparagus in a microwaveable casserole or a glass pie plate. Add a couple of tablespoons water, cover (use plastic wrap or a plate to cover a pie plate), and microwave on High for 3 to 4 minutes.

While the asparagus is cooking, stir the garlic into the olive oil.

When the asparagus is done, drain it. If you have 4 single-serving ovenproof dishes that are large enough to hold asparagus, they're ideal for this purpose—divide the asparagus between the 4 dishes. If not, you'll need to use a rectangular glass baking dish. Arrange the asparagus in 4 groups in the baking dish, like little stacks of cordwood.

Whether you're using the individual dishes or the single baking dish long enough to hold asparagus, drizzle each serving of asparagus with the garlic and olive oil. Salt and pepper lightly, and divide the cheese between the servings. Put the asparagus under the broiler, about 4 inches (10 cm) from low heat. It'll need maybe 4 to 5 minutes. When the Parmesan cheese is touched with gold, serve.

Yield: 4 servings, each with 3 grams of carbohydrates and 1 gram of fiber, for a total of 2 grams of usable carbs and 6 grams of protein.

☉ Simple Grilled Asparagus

Something about the grilling process accentuates the flavor of this dish.
Feel free to do this over your outdoor grill in the summer, by the way.

> 1 pound asparagus (500 g)
>
> 2 to 3 tablespoons olive oil (30 to 50 ml)
>
> Salt and pepper

Preheat your electric tabletop grill.

Snap the ends off the asparagus spears where they break naturally. Place the asparagus on a large plate, drizzle the olive oil over it, then turn it all about with clean hands, so each spear is coated with olive oil. Salt and pepper it.

Lay the asparagus on your grill. How much will fit at once will depend on how big a grill you have; mine will fit most of a pound (500 g). Let it cook for 5 to 6 minutes, then serve.

Yield: 4 servings, each with 3 grams of carbohydrates and 1 gram of fiber, for a total of 2 grams of usable carbs and 1 gram of protein.

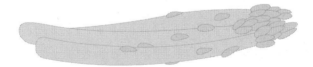

☉ Asparagus Bacon Bundles

Tastes great and has a cool-looking presentation, to boot!

> 1 pound pencil-thin asparagus (500 g)
>
> 7 slices bacon

Preheat your electric tabletop grill.

Snap the ends off the asparagus spears where they break naturally. Divide the asparagus into 7 bunches, and wrap a slice of bacon in a spiral around each bunch. (In other words, don't let the bacon overlap itself, but cover as much of the asparagus bundle as you can.)

Place the asparagus-bacon bundles on the grill. How many will fit will depend on how big your grill is; mine will just fit all 7. Close the grill and let them cook for 7 minutes, or until the bacon is done through, and serve.

Yield: 7 servings, each with 2 grams of carbohydrates and 1 gram of fiber, for a total of 1 gram of usable carbs and 3 grams of protein.

☉ Blue Slaw

A really unusual twist on slaw.

> 4 cups bagged coleslaw mix (300 g)
>
> 3 tablespoons plain yogurt
>
> 1 tablespoon sour cream
>
> 1/4 cup mayonnaise (50 ml)
>
> 2 tablespoons crumbled blue cheese

Just mix everything together—that's all!

Yield: 4 or 5 servings. Assuming 4 servings, each will have 5 grams of carbohydrates and 2 grams of fiber, for a total of 3 grams of usable carbs and 3 grams of protein.

Note: If you want, you can streamline this further by substituting 1/2 cup (100 ml) bottled blue cheese dressing, but it's likely to have a little added sugar. Not much, but a little.

☺ Orange Green Salad

This one's good with anything Mexican or Southwestern in flavor.

8 ounces bagged mixed greens—I like half romaine,
  half red leaf lettuce (250 g)

8 tablespoons chopped cilantro

1/4 sweet red onion, thinly sliced

2 tablespoons orange juice

2 tablespoons white wine vinegar

1/4 teaspoon minced garlic or 1/2 clove garlic, crushed

1/4 teaspoon ground cumin

4 tablespoons oil—a bland oil like canola or peanut is best for this

Put the greens, cilantro, and onion in a large salad bowl. Mix together the juice, vinegar, garlic, and cumin, and set it aside. Pour the oil over the salad and toss well, until all the greens are coated. Pour in the orange juice mixture, toss again, and serve.

Yield: 4 servings, each with 6 grams of carbohydrates and 2 grams of fiber, for a total of 4 grams of usable carbs and 2 grams of protein.

◔ Vegetables Vinaigrette

If your grocery store carries frozen mixed stir-fry peppers with onions, they're a handy item to have in the house. This is gorgeous—and tasty, too. A great choice for a dinner party.

> 1 pound asparagus (500 g)
>
> 3 tablespoons olive oil
>
> 1-pound bag frozen mixed stir-fry peppers with onions, thawed (500 g)
>
> 1/3 cup Italian vinaigrette dressing (70 ml)

Snap the ends off of the asparagus spears where they break naturally. Slice them diagonally into 1/2-inch (1-cm) lengths.

Heat the oil in a large, heavy skillet or wok over high heat. Add the asparagus and stir-fry for 1 to 2 minutes. Add the peppers, and continue stir-frying until the vegetables are tender-crisp. Stir in the dressing, let the whole thing cook for another minute, and serve.

Yield: 6 to 8 servings. Assuming 8 servings, each will have 7 grams of carbohydrates and 2 grams of fiber, for a total of 5 grams of usable carbs and 1 gram of protein.

☺ Orange Pecan Sprouts

My husband took a bite of these, pointed to his plate, and said, "You could make these again!" Really wonderful.

> 1 pound brussels sprouts (500 g)
>
> 1/3 cup chopped pecans (30 g)
>
> 3 tablespoons butter
>
> 1 teaspoon grated orange zest
>
> 3 tablespoons orange juice

Trim the stems of the Brussels sprouts and remove any wilted outer leaves. Run the sprouts through the slicing blade of your food processor.

In a large, heavy skillet over medium-high heat, start sautéing the pecans in the butter. After about 2 minutes, add the Brussels sprouts and sauté the two together, stirring every few minutes until the sprouts soften and start to have a few brown spots. While they're sautéing, you can grate the orange zest and squeeze the orange juice. (You could use bottled orange juice, but since you need the zest, too, fresh just makes sense.) When the sprouts are tender and flecked with brown, stir in the zest and juice, cook for just another minute, and serve.

Yield: 4 servings, each with 12 grams of carbohydrates and 5 grams of fiber, for a total of 7 grams of usable carbs and 4 grams of protein.

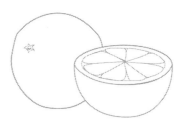

☻ Cumin Mushrooms

A simply amazing accompaniment to the Many-Pepper Steak (see page 110). Also a killer omelet filling (see page 32).

        8 ounces sliced mushrooms (250 g)

        1 1/2 tablespoons butter

        1 1/2 tablespoons olive oil

        1 teaspoon ground cumin

        1/4 teaspoon pepper

        2 tablespoons sour cream

Start sautéing the mushrooms in the butter and oil over medium-high heat. When they've gone limp and changed color, stir in the cumin and pepper. Let the mushrooms cook with the spices for a minute or two, then stir in the sour cream, cook just long enough to heat through, and serve.

Yield: 3 or 4 servings. Assuming 3 servings, each will have 4 grams of carbohydrates and 1 gram of fiber, for a total of 3 grams of usable carbs and 2 grams of protein.

☺ Mushrooms with Bacon, Sun Dried Tomatoes, and Cheese

Just looking at the ingredients in the title, you know you'll love this!

4 slices bacon

8 ounces sliced mushrooms (250 g)

1/2 teaspoon minced garlic or 1 clove fresh garlic

1/4 cup diced sun-dried tomatoes—about 10 pieces before dicing (30 g)

2 tablespoons heavy cream (30 ml)

1/3 cup shredded Parmesan cheese (50 g)

Chop up the bacon or snip it up with kitchen shears. Start cooking it in a large, heavy skillet over medium-high heat. As some grease starts to cook out of the bacon, stir in the mushrooms.

Let the mushrooms cook until they start to change color and get soft. Stir in the garlic and cook for 4 to 5 more minutes. Stir in the tomatoes and cream, and cook until the cream is absorbed. Scatter the cheese over the whole thing, stir it in, let it cook for just another minute, and serve.

Yield: 3 or 4 servings. Assuming 4 servings, each will have 5 grams of carbohydrates and 1 gram of fiber, for a total of 4 grams of usable carbs and 6 grams of protein.

☺ Briar Rose's Artichoke Salad

A cyberpal with the screen name Briar Rose suggested this combination of ingredients to me, and it sounded so phenomenal I just had to play with it. Extraordinary! I was hard-pressed to know whether to call this a side dish or a main dish salad—it's in the in-between range, protein-wise. Call it a substantial side dish or a light meal.

1 can (13.75 ounces, 400 g) quartered artichoke hearts, drained and coarsely chopped

2 ounces sliced pepperoni, sliced into 1/4-inch strips (50 g)

1/4 cup chopped sweet red onion* (30 g)

2 tablespoons chopped fresh basil

1/2 cup crumbled Gorgonzola (50 g)

3 tablespoons extra-virgin olive oil

1/2 teaspoon minced garlic or1 clove garlic, crushed

1 1/2 tablespoons balsamic vinegar

* Actually, Briar Rose doesn't like this, so leave it out if you want to. I'm hopelessly devoted to red onion.

Simply mix everything together and stir well. That's it!

I like to serve this on a bed of lettuce, but it's remarkably good right out of the mixing bowl. For that matter, you could toss it with lettuce that's been broken up well or with bagged mixed greens. Oh, heck, it's hard to think of a bad way to serve this!

Yield: 3 servings, each with 11 grams of carbohydrates and 1 gram of fiber, for a total of 10 grams of usable carbs (though quite a lot of that is a carbohydrate called "inulin," found in artichokes, which has the lowest blood sugar impact of any carbohydrate yet identified, so this is actually a lot easier on your body than the carb count suggests) and 11 grams of protein.

Tip: To save time, stack up the pepperoni rounds and slice them several at a time.

Note: Gorgonzola is the Italian version of blue cheese (although the veins are actually greenish). It's a little milder and creamier than a lot of blue cheeses, and it's quite delicious. However, if you can't find Gorgonzola, feel free to substitute your favorite blue cheese.

☺ Country-Style Green Beans

Okay, truly country-style green beans are cooked for a billion hours with bacon or a ham hock, but that hardly makes for a 15-minute recipe, now does it? And this version tastes very good and down-home.

> 1 pound frozen "cut" green beans (500 g)
>
> 3 slices bacon
>
> 4 ounces sliced mushrooms (120 g)
>
> 1/2 tablespoon butter
>
> 1 tablespoon lemon juice

Put the beans in a microwaveable casserole with a lid, add a couple of tablespoons of water, cover, and microwave on High for 7 minutes.

Cut the bacon into little pieces and put it in a large, heavy skillet—I use kitchen shears to snip it right into the pan—and start cooking it over medium-high heat. When a little grease starts to cook out of the bacon, add the mushrooms and butter, and cook it all together, stirring frequently, until the bacon is starting to get crispy and the mushrooms have softened and changed color.

Somewhere during this process, your microwave is going to go "ding!" When it does, go check the beans. Chances are they'll still be underdone in the center, so stir them up and give them another 4 to 5 minutes.

When the beans are tender-crisp, pull them out of the microwave, drain them, and stir them into the bacon and mushrooms. Stir in the lemon juice, let the whole thing cook together for just another minute or two to combine the flavors, then serve.

Yield: 4 or 5 servings. Assuming 4 servings, each will have 10 grams of carbohydrates and 4 grams of fiber, for a total of 6 grams of usable carbs and 4 grams of protein.

⊕ Apple Walnut Dressing

This dressing has no grain of any kind in it, and still tastes great. Serve with a simple poultry or pork dish.

> 4 tablespoons butter
>
> 1 crisp, tart apple (I use a Granny Smith because I like the flavor, but one with a red skin would look prettier)
>
> 2 large stalks celery
>
> 1 medium onion
>
> 1 cup shelled walnuts (100 g)
>
> 8 ounces sliced mushrooms (250 g)
>
> 3/4 teaspoon salt or Vege-Sal
>
> 1 1/2 teaspoons poultry seasoning

Melt the butter in a large, heavy skillet over medium heat.

Quarter the apple and trim out the core, whack each quarter in half (making eighths), and drop them in your food processor with the S-blade in place. Whack each stalk of celery into 4 or 5 big chunks and throw them in, too. Quarter the onion, peel it, and throw it in, and then dump in the walnuts. Pulse the food processor until everything's a medium consistency.

Dump this mixture, along with the mushrooms (which we're assuming you bought already sliced—if not, just chop 'em with everything else), into the butter in the skillet, turn the heat up to medium-high, and sauté everything for a minute or two, stirring. Then cover it and let it cook for 10 minutes, uncovering every 3 minutes or so to stir the whole thing again.

Stir in the salt and poultry seasoning, let it cook for another minute or two, and serve.

Yield: 6 to 8 servings. Assuming 6 servings, each will have 9 grams of carbohydrates and 3 grams of fiber, for a total of 6 grams of usable carbs and 6 grams of protein.

Regarding Bagged Salad

There are now approximately 482 varieties of bagged salad available in your average grocery store, and what a fine development that is. For once we have a packaged food that is as good for us as it is convenient, sing Glory Hallelujah!

Do yourself a favor and venture beyond the standard Iceberg Mix or American Blend. Iceberg is the least nutritious of the lettuces and the blandest, as well. If you buy bagged salad, try a new blend at least once every couple of weeks, to find out what you might have been missing.

You'll probably be buying bottled salad dressing, too. Remember that the fat-free dressings virtually always have a lot of added sugar! So, too, does any dressing that tastes sweet—Russian, Catalina, that red stuff that calls itself "French," Poppyseed, Honey Mustard, Raspberry Vinaigrette. All are likely culprits, so read the labels carefully.

Overall, you can trust most of the following dressings in their full-fat versions: Blue Cheese (occasionally called Roquefort), Caesar, Creamy Garlic, Red Wine Vinaigrette, Italian, Ranch, Parmesan Peppercorn. However, read the labels to find the brands with the lowest sugar content.

Here's an unsolicited plug: I love Paul Newman's salad dressings. At this writing, I have his Original Olive Oil and Vinegar, Caesar, and Balsamic Vinaigrette in the house, and I think they're all terrific. If you buy the full-fat versions of Paul's dressings they tend to be lower carb than similar dressings in other brands, and they contain no junk chemicals. Good stuff; look for them.

Now, bagged greens with bottled dressings are all well and good, but sometimes you want something more in your salads. I trust you're clear on the idea of adding some diced green pepper, sliced cucumber, some sliced scallions or sweet onion, a radish or two, or a few cherry tomatoes, but what if you want some crunch to replace the croutons? Try:

Sunflower seeds.

Pumpkin seeds. Under the name "Pumpkorn," roasted and flavored pumpkin seeds in many flavors are becoming more and more widely available, or are available online. Pick one to go with your menu.

Diced or broken pork rinds.

Sliced, toasted, flavored almonds. Sunkist recently started distributing these under the name "Almond Accents." They're very crisp and tasty, and they come in a neat variety of flavors, including Roasted Garlic Caesar, Italian

Parmesan, Bacon Cheddar, Garlic Teriyaki, Ranch, and Nacho Cheese. Look for them in the produce aisle of big grocery stores. These make a nice snack, too.

Crumbled bacon. I can't abide fake bacon bits, nor do I like the real bacon bits in a jar—they're soggy and flat-tasting, if you ask me. But it's not much work to throw a few slices of bacon into a glass pie plate, microwave them on High for a few minutes, and then crumble them up. (In most microwaves, about 1 minute per slice is about right, but you'll have to play with your microwave to know for sure.)

Crunchy cheesy bits. If you're used to putting shredded cheddar or the like on your salads, try this: Spray a microwaveable plate with nonstick cooking spray and throw a good handful of cheese—cheddar, Monterey Jack, Parmesan, or any natural, unprocessed hard cheese—on it. Use maybe 1/3 to 1/2 cup (around 50 g). Microwave on High for 1 minute. (The time may vary a bit, depending on your microwave.) It will melt into a disc that will be crispy as it cools. Crumble it over your salad for crunchy, crouton-like bits that have all the full flavor of cheese! This also makes a great snack.

Another thing to consider on busy nights is foregoing salad in favor of cut-up vegetables with dip. One real benefit of this is that—according to my sister Kim, The World's Best Second Grade Teacher—children will eat virtually anything if you give them Ranch dressing to dip it in. Put out a plate of celery sticks, pepper strips, cut-up broccoli and cauliflower, and some baby carrots (which you'll go easy on, right?), along with a bowl of Ranch dressing while you're getting the rest of the meal on the table. You know—do this while the family is starved and looking for something to eat right now. You may be surprised how many vegetables you can get into them this way (especially if you hide the chips), and with almost no work.

Regarding the Virtues of the Salad Bar

Salad bars aren't as common in grocery stores as they were 10 to 12 years back, which is a darn shame—but you can still find grocery stores that have these exceedingly useful features. If you're a reluctant cook, it is worth your while to seek out a local grocery store that does have a salad bar.

Why? Well, obviously it will let you make salads easily. But more than that, it's a great source of prepared ingredients. Use chopped onions a lot? Buy a container of pre-chopped onions from the salad bar, enough for 3 or 4 days, and stash 'em in the fridge. Need sliced peppers for a stir-fry? Hit the salad bar! Heck, I remember being at the salad bar at Sunset Foods in Highland Park, Illinois, on the day before Thanksgiving many years ago, and watching all the local women buying the onions and celery and such for their turkey stuffing. I was dumbstruck with admiration for their cleverness.

So check out the local salad bar, and see what pre-prepped ingredients it offers you!

Regarding Plain Cooked Vegetables

When you're in a hurry and in the mood for a simple, plain cooked vegetable, you have a couple of choices. Fresh vegetables, although wonderful, will generally be the most work, although you can find some of them (most notably broccoli and cauliflower) cut up and ready to cook in your grocery store's produce section. But if you're trying to do minimal cooking, you probably won't want to take the time to, say, top and tail a whole pound (500 g) of green beans, or trim the stems and leaves of several dozen Brussels sprouts.

This leaves you with canned or frozen. Personally, I much prefer frozen vegetables. I consider them superior to canned both in taste and texture, not to mention nutrition. (The canned-good manufacturers insist that canned vegetables are just as good, nutritionally, as frozen or fresh. This is apparently so—provided you consume all the water in the can, and who ever does that, except when making soup?) I'd go with the frozen vegetables, of which your grocery store freezer section has an ever-expanding variety.

The most important thing to know about frozen vegetables is the fastest, easiest way to cook them to get superior results, both for eating quality and nutrition. That method is microwaving. You've probably noticed the repeated use of the microwave in the recipes here. This is because the microwave is one of the very best ways to cook vegetables, yielding results that are better than boiling or steaming vegetables on the stove, and—because very little water is used—retaining more vitamins, too. Almost all frozen vegetables now come with microwave instructions on the package. Use them!

Another important tip: No matter what method you use to cook your vegetables, when they are done to your taste, uncover them. Do not keep the lid on them while you finish preparing the rest of the meal. I know you're just trying to keep them warm, but what you're actually doing is letting them continue cooking. That's how they end up gray and mushy and icky, and your kids grow up hating vegetables. Better to remove the lid to let out the steam, and then—if the rest of dinner is going to take another 5 to 10 minutes—put the lid back on, leaving a 1/2-inch (1 cm) crack. This will hold in heat without overcooking your veggies. If the meal is seriously delayed, you can always reheat your vegetables for a minute or two, which is a lot better than cooking them to a pulp.

You'll serve your veggies with butter and a little salt and pepper, no doubt, but don't forget that there are easy things to do with vegetables, too. A little lemon juice is wonderful on many vegetables, especially broccoli and green beans. Garlic is good, too, and you can buy garlic-infused olive oil to drizzle over vegetables to great effect. (You can also make your own by putting a few cloves of crushed garlic or a few teaspoons of jarred, minced garlic in a squeeze bottle and filling it with olive oil.) Lemon-pepper is good on many veggies, and how about Cajun seasoning? It doesn't take a lot of work to do something a little different and good, it just takes remembering to do it.

chapter eleven

15-Minute Soups

Of course, to keep within our 15-minute time limit, we won't be making slow-simmered soups. But I think you'll be surprised at just how good a soup you can make in so little time. One word of advice: Do buy the best-quality canned or boxed broth you can get. It makes a big difference.

☺ Cream of Salmon Soup

One person who sampled this soup pronounced it the best soup they'd ever had. And it's so easy!

> 1 1/2 tablespoons butter
> 1/4 cup finely minced onion (30 g)
> 1/4 cup finely minced celery (30 g)
> 2 cups heavy cream (500 ml)
> 14-ounce can salmon, drained (400 g)
> 1/2 teaspoon dried thyme

In a heavy saucepan, melt the butter over medium-low heat, and add the onion and celery. Sauté the vegetables for a few minutes, until the onion is turning translucent.

Meanwhile, pour the cream into a glass 2-cup (500 ml) measure, or any other microwavable container big enough for it and from which you can pour. Place it in the microwave and heat it at 50 percent power for 3 to 4 minutes. (This just cuts the time needed to heat the cream through—you can skip this step and simply heat the soup on the stove top a little longer, if you like.)

Pour the cream into the saucepan, and add the salmon and thyme. Break up the salmon as you stir the soup—I found my whisk to be ideal for breaking the salmon into fine pieces. Heat until simmering, and serve.

Yield: 4 servings, each with 5 grams of carbohydrates, a trace of fiber, and 23 grams of protein.

☺ Mexican Cabbage Soup

Great on a nasty, cold, rainy night! This is not hot, despite the chilies in the canned tomatoes—feel free to pass the hot sauce at the table if you want to spice it up. With all these vegetables, this is a complete meal, but if the family insists, you could add some corn tortillas for them.

>   1 quart beef broth (1 l)
>   14-ounce can diced tomatoes with green chilies (400 g)
>   1 pound ground round or other very lean ground beef (500 g)
>   1 tablespoon oil
>   ¹/₂ cup chopped onion (50 g)
>   1 teaspoon minced garlic or 2 cloves garlic, crushed
>   1 teaspoon ground cumin
>   2 teaspoons oregano
>   2 cups bagged coleslaw mix (150 g)

In a large, microwaveable container combine the beef broth and canned tomatoes. Microwave on High for 8 to 10 minutes.

While the broth and tomatoes are heating through, start browning and crumbling the beef in the oil. Use a large soup kettle or heavy-bottomed saucepan. When the beef's about half browned, add the onion and garlic. Continue cooking until the beef is entirely browned. Add the cumin and oregano, and stir them in, then add the heated beef stock and tomatoes. Stir in the coleslaw mix and bring the whole thing to a simmer. Cook for another minute or so, and serve.

Yield: 4 servings, each with 9 grams of carbohydrates and 2 grams of fiber, for a total of 7 grams of usable carbs and 24 grams of protein.

☉ Oyster Stew

A classic recipe that simply started out fast, easy, and low-carb. My husband prefers me to cut really big oysters into quarters. Since you can do this as the cream and half-and-half are heating, it doesn't add any time to the recipe—indeed, since the pieces of oyster cook faster than whole ones, it cuts the cooking time a bit.

> 5 tablespoons butter (75 ml)
>
> 1 cup half-and-half (250 ml)
>
> 1 1/2 cups heavy cream (350 ml)
>
> 1/2 cup water (120 ml)
>
> 1 1/2 pints oysters (700 g)
>
> Salt and pepper
>
> 1/8 teaspoon cayenne

Put the butter, half-and-half, heavy cream, and water in a heavy-bottomed saucepan over medium heat. As it comes to a simmer, add the oysters, and stir. Simmer until the oysters are cooked, about 5 minutes. Salt and pepper to taste, add the cayenne, then serve.

Yield: 4 servings, each with 8 grams of carbohydrates, no fiber, and 11 grams of protein. Despite the modest protein count, this is filling because it is so rich.

Note: If you'd like to speed this recipe up, you can combine everything but the oysters in a good-size microwaveable container and nuke it for 5 minutes on High, but it's not essential.

☉ Stir-Fry Soup

The name says it all—a traditional stir-fry turned into a hearty soup. This works equally well with chicken or pork, so take your pick or use whatever is cluttering up the freezer.

> 2 quarts chicken broth (2 l)
> 1 pound boneless pork loin (500 g) or 1 pound boneless, skinless
>   chicken breast (500 g)
> 1 medium onion
> 3 tablespoons oil
> 1-pound bag frozen stir-fry vegetables, thawed (500 g)
> 1 1/2 tablespoons soy sauce
> 1 1/2 tablespoons dry sherry
> 1 1/2 tablespoons grated gingerroot
> 1 1/2 teaspoons minced garlic
> 1 1/2 teaspoons toasted sesame oil

Pour the chicken broth into a large microwaveable bowl or pitcher. Put it in the microwave and nuke it for 10 minutes on High.

Slice the pork or chicken as thin as possible. (This is easier if the meat is partly frozen.) Thinly slice the onion, as well. Heat the oil in the bottom of a large soup kettle, and add the meat, onion, and stir-fry vegetables. Stir-fry everything over highest heat while the broth is warming in the microwave.

By the time the microwave goes "ding," the pork or chicken should not be pink anymore. Pour in the broth, add the soy sauce, sherry, gingerroot, garlic, and sesame oil, cover, and let the whole thing simmer for 4 to 5 minutes before serving.

Yield: 6 servings, each with 9 grams of carbohydrates and 2 grams of fiber, for a total of 7 grams of usable carbs and 19 grams of protein.

⊕ Italian Sausage Soup

This takes some serious multi-tasking to get done in 15 minutes, but it was too good not to include.

> 1 1/2 quarts chicken broth (1.5 l)
>
> 1-pound bag frozen Italian Vegetable Blend (500 g)
>
> 1 pound Italian sausage, mild or hot, as you prefer (500 g)
>
> 1/2 medium onion, chopped
>
> 1 teaspoon minced garlic or 2 cloves garlic, crushed
>
> 2 teaspoons Italian seasoning
>
> 3 eggs
>
> 5 tablespoons grated or shredded Parmesan cheese

First, put the broth in a good-size saucepan, cover it, and place it over high heat. Next, put the Italian Vegetable Blend in a microwaveable casserole, add a couple of tablespoons of water, cover, and microwave on High for 12 minutes.

Okay, that stuff is under control. Now, in a heavy-bottomed kettle, start browning the Italian sausage over medium-high heat. If the sausage is in links, slit the skins and squeeze it out, so you can crumble it; bulk sausage you can just plunk into the kettle. As a bit of grease starts to cook out of the sausage, add the onion and the garlic (you can chop the onion while the sausage is browning), and let them sauté together.

When the sausage is cooked through, add the chicken broth, which should be hot by now. Stir, and add the Italian seasoning. Let the mixture simmer while you crack the eggs into a glass measuring cup and beat them with a fork. Pour the eggs in, a little bit at a time—pour, then stir, pour some more, then stir some more. This will make lovely egg shreds in your soup.

The vegetables should be done by now, so pull them out of the microwave, drain, and dump them into the soup. Stir, let the whole thing simmer for just another minute, and serve with a tablespoon of Parmesan cheese on each serving.

Yield: 5 servings, each with 11 grams of carbohydrates and 2 grams of fiber, for a total of 9 grams of usable carbs and 26 grams of protein.

⊕ Pantry Seafood Bisque

Quick, easy, tasty, and what a gorgeous pale pink color! Simple to double, of course, but it'll take a little longer for the larger quantity of half-and-half to heat through. You could microwave it to speed things along, if you like.

> 1 pint half-and-half (500 ml)
>
> 3 tablespoons tomato paste
>
> 1 can (4 ounces) tiny shrimp, drained (120 g)
>
> 1 can (6 ounces) flaked crab, drained (170 g)
>
> 1 teaspoon dried dill weed
>
> 1/2 teaspoon lemon juice
>
> Salt and pepper to taste

In a largish saucepan over low heat, heat the half-and-half to just below a simmer. Whisk in the tomato paste, then stir in the shrimp, crab, dill, and lemon juice. Let the whole thing cook together for just a minute or two, salt and pepper to taste, and serve.

Yield: 3 servings, each with 11 grams of carbohydrates and 1 gram of fiber, for a total of 10 grams of usable carbs and 24 grams of protein.

✻ Each serving also has 254 milligrams of calcium!

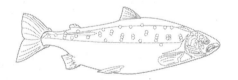

☉ Almost Lobster Bisque

Monkfish has long been known as "poor man's lobster," so I decided to use it in a classic lobster bisque. However, if your budget allows, feel free to use lobster tail in this recipe instead.

> 1/2 cup heavy cream (120 ml)
>
> 1 cup half-and-half (250 ml)
>
> 1/2 cup water (120 ml)
>
> 10 ounce monkfish fillet (300 g)
>
> 1/2 cup dry sherry (120 ml)
>
> 1 1/2 teaspoons Dana's No-Sugar Ketchup (see page 224)
>   or other sugar-free ketchup
>
> 1/2 teaspoon Worcestershire sauce
>
> 1/2 teaspoon lemon juice
>
> 1/2 teaspoon salt or Vege-Sal
>
> Guar or xanthan (optional)
>
> 1 scallion, finely sliced

First combine the cream, half-and-half, and water in a large, microwaveable dish. Microwave for 5 to 6 minutes on 70 percent power.

While the cream is heating, cut the monkfish fillet into bite-size pieces. Bring the sherry to a simmer in a large, heavy-bottomed saucepan over medium-high heat. Add the monkfish, turn the burner down a touch, and let the fish simmer in the sherry, stirring occasionally, for 4 to 5 minutes, or until cooked through.

Stir in the cream, which should be hot by now. Stir in the ketchup, Worcestershire sauce, lemon juice, and salt, and heat it only to a simmer. If you'd like your bisque thicker, feel free to use guar or xanthan, but it's mighty nice the way it is. Ladle into dishes, and top each serving with a scattering of sliced scallion.

Yield: 2 servings, each with 10 grams of carbohydrates, a trace of fiber, and 26 grams of protein.

⊕ Instant Chicken Soup

Okay, so this isn't quite as instant as those little packets you mix with boiling water. But it's a lot tastier, a lot heartier, and a lot better for you.

 ¹/₄ head cauliflower

 1 quart, or two 14.5-ounce cans, chicken broth (1 l)

 10 to 12 ounces boneless, skinless chicken breast (350 g)

 1 stalk celery

 1 medium carrot

 ¹/₄ medium onion

 1 tablespoon butter

 1 ¹/₂ teaspoons poultry seasoning

 Salt and pepper

Run the cauliflower through the shredding blade of your food processor. Put it in a microwaveable bowl, add a tablespoon of water, cover, and microwave on High for 5 minutes.

While that's cooking, pour the broth into a large saucepan over high heat. Dice the chicken breast into small bits—about ¹/₂-inch (1 cm) cubes—and add it to the pot.

Take the shredding disc out of the food processor, put the S-blade in place, and put the celery, carrot, and onion, cut into a few big hunks, in the food processor bowl. Pulse to chop to a medium-fine consistency.

Melt the butter in a medium-size heavy skillet over medium-high heat, and add the vegetables and the poultry seasoning. Sauté, stirring frequently.

When the microwave goes "ding," pull the cauliflower out of the microwave and add it to the soup. You can add the other veggies straight from the skillet or, if you'd like them to be a little softer, put them in the bowl you cooked the cauliflower in, add a tablespoon of the broth from the soup, cover, and microwave them for 3 to 4 minutes on High before adding them to the soup.

Either way, stir the vegetables into the soup, salt and pepper to taste, and serve.

Yield: 3 or 4 servings. Assuming 3 servings, each will have 6 grams of carbohydrates and 1 gram of fiber, for a total of 5 grams of usable carbs and 28 grams of protein.

Note: If you'd prefer, you can make this with egg threads instead of the cauliflower rice, and it will be higher in protein. Just beat a couple of eggs in a measuring cup and pour the beaten egg over the simmering soup, stirring slowly with a fork.

☉ Cheater's Chowder

So called because you're cheating on the usual ingredients, and you sure are cheating on the cooking time! You are not, however, cheating on your diet. This filling soup is a meal in itself.

> 1/4 head cauliflower
>
> 1 medium turnip (just bigger than a tennis ball)
>
> 3 slices bacon
>
> 1/2 medium onion
>
> 2 cups half-and-half (500 ml)
>
> 10-ounce can minced clams (300 g)
>
> Salt or Vege-Sal and pepper

Whack the cauliflower into a few good-size chunks, and put it in your food processor with the S-blade in place. Peel the turnip, quarter it, and drop it in there, too. Pulse the processor until everything's chopped to a medium-fine consistency. Put the cauliflower and turnip in a microwaveable casserole with a lid, add a couple of tablespoons of water, cover, and microwave on High for 12 minutes.

While that's cooking, chop up the bacon (I snip mine up with cooking shears, right into the pot) and start frying it over medium-high heat in a large, heavy-bottomed saucepan, stirring from time to time.

Put that food processor bowl back on its base with the S-blade in place, throw in the half-onion, and pulse until the onion's chopped medium-fine. Dump the onion in with the bacon, which should be giving off some grease by now. Fry the onion and bacon together until the onion is translucent.

Pour the half-and-half and the clams into the pot—don't bother to drain the clams —stir it, and then let the whole thing come to a simmer, stirring from time to time.

When the cauliflower and turnips are done, add them to the pot, too—no need to drain. Stir them in, salt and pepper it to taste, let the soup simmer just another minute or two, and serve.

Yield: 3 servings, each with 16 grams of carbohydrates and 1 gram of fiber, for a total of 15 grams of usable carbs and 31 grams of protein.

By the way, I tried running the nutritional analysis for this soup using half heavy cream in place of the half-and-half. It only cut 1 gram of carb off each serving— but it added 175 calories. Not worth it, if you ask me.

☺ Sopa Aguacate

With one of the quesadillas from Chapter Two on the side (see page 51), this makes a nice light supper.

> 1 quart chicken broth (1 l)
>
> 1 ripe avocado
>
> 2 scallions
>
> 2 canned green chilies or 1 or 2 canned jalapeños, if you like it hot!
>
> 2 tablespoons chopped cilantro
>
> 1/2 teaspoon salt or Vege-Sal

Start heating the broth—you can put it in a pan on the stove, or you can put it in a large microwaveable container in the microwave.

While the broth is heating, scoop the avocado out of its skin and into a food processor with the S-blade in place. Add the scallions, peppers, cilantro, and salt. Pulse to chop everything together—you can leave a few chunks of avocado or purée it smooth, whichever you prefer.

When the broth is hot, divide the avocado mixture between 4 smallish soup bowls. Ladle the hot broth over the avocado mixture, and serve.

Yield: 4 servings, each with 6 grams of carbohydrates and 3 grams of fiber, for a total of 3 grams of usable carbs and 6 grams of protein.

Bonus: You'll get a whopping 572 mgs potassium and only 125 calories!

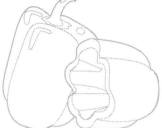

chapter twelve

15-Minute Condiments, Sauces, Dressings, and Seasonings

When you read the labels, you'll be stunned at how much sugar you'll find in condiments, sauces, salad dressings, and even some sprinkle-on seasonings. Fortunately, it's quite quick and simple to make your own.

Many of these condiments, sauces, dressings, and seasonings are called for in other recipes in the book. Others are not but are included because they offer great, easy ways to season the simple slabs of protein—chicken breasts, fish fillets, steaks, chops, and so on—that are the staples of quick low-carb cooking.

You'll find some new recipes here, plus a few I've repeated from *500 Low-Carb Recipes*—the ones I thought would be most helpful for making quick and varied meals.

Dipping Sauces

Dipping sauces are an increasingly popular way to add variety to simple foods—even McDonald's offers dipping sauces with their McNuggets! Each of these dipping sauces is called for in another recipe in this book, but feel free to use them any way you like.

☺ "Honey" Mustard Dipping Sauce

Great with the fried Chicken Tenders (see page 72) or with a simple chicken breast or pork chop.

> 1/4 cup mayonnaise (50 ml)
>
> 2 tablespoons spicy mustard
>
> 1 teaspoon Splenda

Simply combine everything, and you're all set.

Yield: Makes a little more than 1/3 cup (about 70 ml), or enough for about 4 people eating Chicken Tenders. Each serving has 1 gram of carbohydrates, no fiber, and 1 gram of protein.

☺ Apricot Ginger Dipping Sauce

Also great with Chicken Tenders (see page 72)—or anything else you might use the "Honey" Mustard Dipping Sauce on—only it tastes a lot different.

> 1/4 cup mayonnaise (50 ml)
>
> 1 1/2 tablespoons low-sugar apricot preserves
>
> 1 teaspoon grated gingerroot
>
> 1/4 teaspoon minced ginger or 1/2 clove garlic, crushed
>
> 1/2 teaspoon Splenda
>
> 3/4 teaspoon soy sauce

Simply combine everything.

Yield: Makes just under 1/3 cup (about 70 ml), or enough for about 4 people eating Chicken Tenders. Each serving has 3 grams of carbohydrates, with a trace of fiber and protein.

☉ Asian Dipping Sauce

Perfect with the Lettuce Wraps on page 81, but also good with Chicken Tenders (see page 72), or whatever you have on hand.

> ¹/₄ cup Splenda (30 g)
>
> ¹/₄ cup water (50 ml)
>
> 2 tablespoons soy sauce
>
> 2 tablespoons rice vinegar
>
> 2 tablespoons Dana's No-Sugar Ketchup (see page 224)
>
>   or commercial sugar-free ketchup
>
> 1 tablespoon lemon juice
>
> ¹/₄ teaspoon toasted sesame oil
>
> 2 teaspoons dry mustard
>
> 2 teaspoons chili garlic paste

Just assemble everything in a blender, and run it until everything's well combined. If you don't use it all up at once, keep in a tightly sealed container in the fridge and it will last a week, at least.

Yield: Makes roughly 3/4 cup (175 ml), or 6 servings of 2 tablespoons each. Each serving has 3 grams of carbohydrates, a trace of fiber, and 1 gram of protein.

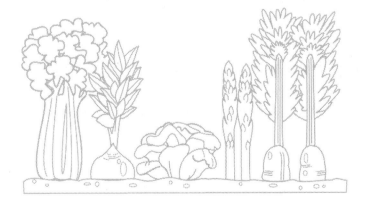

☺ Nuoc Cham

This sweet-tart-spicy dipping sauce is purely Vietnamese, and absolutely wonderful! Essential for the Lemon Chicken (see page 67) and the Vietnamese Chicken Salad (see page 119), but once you try this, you'll think of all sorts of ways to use it.

> 2 tablespoons fish sauce
>
> 2 tablespoons lime juice
>
> 1 1/2 teaspoons rice vinegar
>
> 3 tablespoons Splenda
>
> 1/2 teaspoon minced garlic or 1 clove garlic, crushed
>
> 1 teaspoon chili garlic paste

Simply combine everything in a small dish.

Yield: About 1/3 cup (75 ml), or 4 or 5 servings. Assuming 4 servings, each will have 4 grams of carbohydrates, a trace of fiber, and a trace of protein. (And approximately 15 metric boatloads of flavor!)

☺ Stir-Fry Sauce

If you like Chinese food, make this up and keep it on hand. Then you can just throw any sort of meat and vegetables in your wok or skillet and have a meal in minutes.

> 1/2 cup soy sauce (120 ml)
>
> 1/2 cup dry sherry (120 ml)
>
> 2 cloves garlic, crushed, or 1 teaspoon minced garlic
>
> 2 tablespoons grated fresh ginger
>
> 2 teaspoons Splenda

Simply combine everything, and store in a tightly sealed container in the refrigerator.

Yield: Makes 1 cup (250 ml). Use about 1 1/2 to 2 tablespoons (22 to 30 ml) per serving of stir-fry. Each serving contains 2 grams of carbohydrates, no fiber, and no protein.

☉ Easy Remoulade Sauce

Good on anything fishy or seafoodlike.

>   1 cup mayonnaise (250 ml)
>
>   2 tablespoons spicy brown or Dijon mustard)
>
>   2 tablespoons lemon juice
>
>   1 teaspoon dried tarragon, crumbled
>
>   2 tablespoons capers, drained and chopped a bit

Just stir everything up, and you're good to go!

Yield: Makes about 1 1/3 cups (325 ml), or 5 servings of just under 1/4 cup (50 ml) each. Each serving has 1 gram of carbohydrates, a trace of fiber, and 1 gram of protein.

Salad Dressings

When you're pressed for time or just avoiding cooking, you're likely to use bottled salad dressing. No reason not to, so long as you stick to the low-carb varieties. However, I'm including two salad dressing recipes, the first because it's so unusual and it's used in a few recipes elsewhere in this book, and the second—a repeat from *500 Low-Carb Recipes*—because coleslaw is tremendously popular, yet so often sugary.

☺ Guacamole Dressing

Guacamole thinned out just enough to make a salad dressing—wonderful! Remember, the little black avocados are much lower in carbs than the big green ones. Do use this dressing up pretty quickly; you know how avocado changes color. If you must keep the leftovers for a day, store them in a tightly sealed container in the refrigerator.

> 1 ripe avocado
>
> 1/2 cup plain yogurt (120 ml)
>
> 1/4 cup olive oil (50 ml)
>
> 1 tablespoon lime juice
>
> 1/2 teaspoon minced garlic or 1 clove garlic, crushed
>
> 1/4 teaspoon hot sauce
>
> 1/4 teaspoon salt

Cut the avocado in half, remove the seed, and scoop the flesh into a blender or food processor. Add the yogurt, olive oil, lime juice, garlic, hot sauce, and salt, and blend until smooth.

Yield: 4 servings, each with 6 grams of carbohydrates and 2 grams of fiber, for a total of 4 grams of usable carbs (actually less if you use the *GO-Diet's* figure of 4 grams of carbohydrates per cup [225 ml] of plain yogurt) and 3 grams of protein.

✵ A serving of this dressing packs more potassium than a banana!

☺ Coleslaw Dressing

Virtually all commercial coleslaw dressing is simply full of sugar, which is a shame, since cabbage is a very low-carb vegetable. I just love coleslaw, so I had to come up with a sugar-free dressing! Make this up, pour it over a bag or two of pre-shredded coleslaw mix, and you'll have a great, versatile side dish in no time. Always try to make lots of coleslaw; it gets better over the day or two after it's made.

> 1/2 cup mayonnaise (120 ml)
>
> 1/2 cup sour cream (120 ml)
>
> 1 to 1 1/2 tablespoons apple cider vinegar
>
> 1 to 1 1/2 teaspoons prepared mustard
>
> 1/2 to 1 teaspoon salt or Vege-Sal
>
> 1/2 to 1 packet artificial sweetener, or Splenda

Just mix it all together, and you're all set!

Yield: Assuming that you get 12 servings out of a batch, this dressing will add only 1 gram of carbohydrates to each serving, plus a trace of fiber and protein.

Variation: You may, of course, vary these proportions to taste. Also, a teaspoon or so of celery seed can be nice in this. This much would be enough for at least two bags of coleslaw mix, as far as I'm concerned, but use an amount to suit your taste.

Sprinkle-On Seasonings

Sprinkle-on seasonings are a simple way to vary "chicken again, chops again, steak again" and the like. There are many good varieties to choose from in your grocery store, and I urge you to put together a modest collection! However, if you'd like to make your own, they're very little work for a lot of result—plus, when you make sprinkle-on seasonings yourself, you know that they're sugar-free. Here are some I've come up with that I like.

☉ Many-Pepper Steak Seasoning

Adds real zing to a steak without covering up the flavor. Make this up, keep it in a shaker, and you'll be ready to cook a really special steak at a moment's notice.

    1 tablespoon onion powder

    3 tablespoons garlic powder

    3 tablespoons paprika

    1 tablespoon oregano

    1 1/2 tablespoons pepper

    2 teaspoons lemon pepper

    1 teaspoon cayenne—or more if you like it really hot!

Simply combine everything well, and put it in a shaker. Sprinkle liberally over both sides of a steak before broiling or grilling.

Yield: This is enough to season 12 to 15 steaks. Assuming 15 steaks, each will have 3 grams of carbohydrates and 1 gram of fiber, or for a total of 2 grams of carbs to a whole steak—and that steak is likely to be 2 or more servings, so figure 1 gram per serving—and no fiber or protein.

☉ Dana's Chicken Seasoning

This is wonderful sprinkled over a chicken breast before grilling or as a table seasoning for any poultry. (It's also great sprinkled over whole or cut-up chicken before roasting, but that doesn't fit into our 15-minute time frame.)

3 tablespoons salt

1 teaspoon paprika

1 teaspoon onion powder

1 teaspoon garlic powder

1 teaspoon curry powder

1/2 teaspoon black pepper

Combine all the ingredients thoroughly, and store in a salt shaker or the shaker from an old container of herbs. Simply sprinkle over chicken before roasting; I use it to season at the table, as well.

Yield: Makes just over 1/4 cup (30 g). In the whole recipe there are only 7 grams of carbohydrates and 1 gram of fiber, for a total of 6 grams of usable carbs and no protein—so the amount of carbohydrates in the teaspoon or so you sprinkle over a piece of chicken is negligible.

☺ Cajun Seasoning

This sprinkle-on seasoning will liven up chops, steaks, chicken, fish—just about anything!

 2 1/2 tablespoons paprika

 2 tablespoons salt

 2 tablespoons garlic powder

 1 tablespoon black pepper

 1 tablespoon onion powder

 1 tablespoon cayenne pepper

 1 tablespoon dried oregano

 1 tablespoon dried thyme

Combine all the ingredients thoroughly, and keep in an air-tight container.

Yield: Makes 2/3 cup (70 g). In this whole recipe there are 37 grams of carbohydrates and 9 grams of fiber, for a total of 28 grams of usable carbs and no protein. Considering how spicy this is, you're unlikely to use more than a teaspoon or two at a time. One teaspoon has 1 gram of carbohydrates, a trace of fiber, and no protein.

☉ Jerk Seasoning

Sprinkle this over chicken, pork chops, or fish before cooking for an instant hit of hot, sweet, spicy flavor.

  1 tablespoon onion flakes

  2 teaspoons ground thyme

  1 teaspoon ground allspice

  1/4 teaspoon ground cinnamon

  1 teaspoon black pepper

  1 teaspoon cayenne pepper

  1 tablespoon onion powder)

  2 teaspoons salt

  1/4 teaspoon ground nutmeg

  2 tablespoons Splenda

Combine all the ingredients, and store in an air-tight container.

Yield: Makes about 1/3 cup (30 g). If you use 1 teaspoon, it will have 1 gram of carbohydrates, a trace of fiber, and no protein.

☺ Wonderful Memphis-Style Dry Rub BBQ

A *Lowcarbezine!* reader who didn't supply his or her name sent this recipe, so we refer to them simply as the Mystery Chef. This is great on ribs, chops, or chicken, and far lower-carb than barbecue sauce.

> 1 tablespoon paprika
>
> 2 teaspoons chili powder
>
> 3/4 teaspoon salt
>
> 1/4 teaspoon dry mustard
>
> 1/4 teaspoon garlic powder
>
> 1/8 teaspoon pepper

Mix all the ingredients together and store in a salt shaker. Sprinkle on both sides of whatever meat you're cooking, and grill.

Yield: This makes enough for 3 1/2 pounds (1 3/4 kg) of ribs, or about 3 servings. If, indeed, 3 of you eat all of this recipe, each will get 2 grams of carbohydrates and 1 gram of fiber, for a total of 1 gram of usable carbs, no fiber, and no protein. By contrast, your average commercial barbecue sauce has between 10 and 15 grams per 2-tablespoon serving—and who ever stopped at 2 tablespoons?

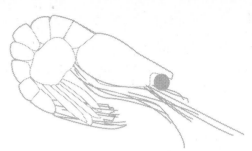

Condiments

Did you know that ketchup has more sugar than ice cream does? You can buy no-sugar ketchup, but it's pricey—and it's not worth it when making your own is such a snap. And once you've got ketchup in the fridge, you can make steak sauce and cocktail sauce. Clearly it is in your best interests to put together a batch of ketchup today!

Commercial barbecue sauce is, I'm sorry to say, even more syrupy than ketchup; so much so that it's very hard to fit most commercial barbecue sauces into your diet. You'll find a recipe for barbecue sauce below, but it's a bit more trouble than the ketchup. There are a few low- or no-sugar barbecue sauces on the market. My favorite is Stubb's, out of Austin, Texas, which has about half the sugar of most commercial barbecue sauces yet tastes at least as good, if not better. It's worth checking your grocery store condiment aisle for it. Walden's is a brand marketed directly to the low-carb market; low-carb e-tailers (online retailers) carry this. I like Stubb's better, but Walden's is lower carb. Atkins also makes a barbecue sauce, but I haven't tried it yet.

☺ Dana's No-Sugar Ketchup

This great-tasting ketchup has all the flavor of your favorite brand, without the high carb count. The guar or xanthan isn't essential, but it makes your ketchup a little thicker and helps keep the water from separating out if you don't use it up quickly.

6-ounce can tomato paste (170 ml)

2/3 cup cider vinegar (150 ml)

1/3 cup water (70 ml)

1/3 cup Splenda (30 g)

2 tablespoons finely minced onion

2 cloves garlic, crushed

1 teaspoon salt or Vege-Sal

1/8 teaspoon ground allspice

1/8 teaspoon ground cloves

1/8 teaspoon pepper

1/4 teaspoon guar or xanthan

Assemble everything in a blender, and run the blender—you'll have to scrape down the sides because this mixture is thick—until the bits of onion disappear. Store in a tightly sealed container in the refrigerator.

Yield: Makes 1 1/2 cups (370 ml) of ketchup, or twenty-four 1-tablespoon servings. Each serving will have 2.25 grams of carbohydrates, a trace of fiber, and a trace of protein.

☐ Low-Carb Steak Sauce

If you have Dana's No-Sugar Ketchup on hand, this is a cinch to make. It's nice to have on hand if you're having a simple broiled steak, and it's indispensable with steak and eggs.

> ¼ cup Dana's No-Sugar Ketchup (50 ml) *see previous page*
>
> 1 tablespoon Worcestershire sauce
>
> 1 teaspoon lemon juice

Simply combine the ingredients well. Store in a tightly sealed container in the refrigerator.

Yield: Makes five 1-tablespoon servings, each with 2.25 grams of carbohydrates, a trace of fiber, and a trace of protein.

☐ Cocktail Sauce

If you like shrimp, frozen, cooked, peeled shrimp are a terrific convenience food—but it's nice to have something to dip them in. Commercial cocktail sauce, like so many other condiments, is full of sugar; you'll save quite a few carbs by making your own.

> ¼ cup Dana's No-Sugar Ketchup (50 m) *see previous page*
>
> 1 teaspoon prepared horseradish

Just stir together, and dip!

Yield: The whole batch has about 9 grams of carbohydrates, a trace of fiber, and no protein.

Note: Mustard and mayonnaise, mixed together, also make a nice dip for shrimp. Or you could buy Dijonnaise. Either way, this mustard-mayo combo is lower in carbs than even the sugar-free cocktail sauce. Try dipping shrimp in Nuoc Cham (see page 214), too.

☉ Reduced-Carb Spicy Barbecue Sauce

Ketchup is bad enough, but barbecue sauce has even more sugar! Make your own. This is, I confess, the only recipe in the book that takes more than 15 minutes—the idea is to have it hanging around in the refrigerator, ready to call on for making Slow Cooker "Barbecued" Ribs (see page 167) and the like. However, if you can find Walden's, Stubb's, or any other reasonably low-carb commercial barbecue sauce, I'll understand if you ignore this recipe.

  1 clove garlic, crushed

  1 small onion, finely minced

  4 tablespoons butter or oil

  4 tablespoons Splenda

  2 teaspoons blackstrap molasses

  1 teaspoon salt or Vege-Sal

  1 teaspoon dry mustard

  1 teaspoon paprika

  1 teaspoon chili powder

  1/2 teaspoon black pepper

  1 1/2 cups water (350 ml)

  1/4 cup cider vinegar (50 ml)

  1 tablespoon Worcestershire sauce

  1 tablespoon prepared horseradish

  1 tablespoon liquid smoke*

  6-ounce can tomato paste (170 ml)

* Most big grocery stores carry this. A company called Colgin makes it.

In a saucepan, cook the onion and garlic in the butter or oil for a few minutes. Stir in the Splenda, molasses, salt, dry mustard, paprika, chili powder, black pepper, water, vinegar, Worcestershire sauce, and horseradish. Let it simmer for 15 to 20 minutes. Then whisk in the tomato paste and smoke flavoring, and let it simmer for another 5 to 10 minutes. Store in a jar in the refrigerator.

Yield: This makes about 2 2/3 cups (600 ml) of sauce, or about twenty-one 2-tablespoon (30 ml) servings, each with 3 grams of carbohydrates and 1 gram of fiber, for a total of 2 grams of usable carbs, no fiber, and no protein.

Marinades

Marinating things, simple though it may be, actually takes us well beyond our 15-minute time limit. So why include these two recipes from *500 Low-Carb Recipes*? Because both of them are good when used in our quick cooking, too. Brushing a little Tequila-Lime Marinade over a chicken breast before sautéing it, then spooning a little more over it as it cooks, adds a lot of flavor. You could also use the Tequila Lime Marinade to flavor sautéed shrimp. As for the Teriyaki Marinade, why not use it with some ribs, chicken, or pork loin in your slow cooker? You'll find a recipe in the slow cooker section where you do exactly that.

☉ Tequila Lime Marinade

Great for boneless, skinless chicken breasts, fish, and shrimp. If you don't have time to marinade, you could pour a little into a skillet while sautéing.

> ¹/₃ cup lime juice, bottled or fresh (70 ml)
>
> ¹/₃ cup water (70 ml)
>
> 3 tablespoon tequila
>
> 1 tablespoon Splenda
>
> 1 tablespoon soy sauce
>
> 2 cloves garlic, crushed

Combine all of the ingredients and refrigerate until use.

Yield: This makes roughly 3/4 cup (170 ml)—enough for a dozen boneless, skinless chicken breasts or a couple of pounds (kilo) of shrimp. The whole batch has 13 grams of carbohydrates and 1 gram of fiber, for a total of 12 grams of usable carbs, no fiber, and no protein. But since you drain most of the marinade off, you won't actually get more than a gram or two of carbs.

◷ Teriyaki Sauce

Good on chicken, beef, fish—just about anything!

   1/2 cup soy sauce (100 ml)

   1/4 cup dry sherry (50 ml)

   1 clove garlic, crushed

   2 tablespoons Splenda

   1 tablespoon grated fresh ginger

Simply combine all of the ingredients and refrigerate until use.

Yield: Makes just over 3/4 cup (170 ml), or almost twelve 1-tablespoon servings, each with about 3 grams of carbohydrates, no fiber, and no protein.

chapter thirteen

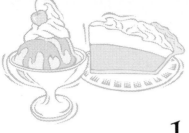

15~Minute Desserts

I didn't put in a lot of work on dessert recipes for this book for a simple reason: If you're scrambling for time and need to get everything on the table as quickly as possible, you're not going to take an extra 15 minutes to make dessert! And if you're the sort of person who simply hates cooking, you're probably going to put your limited efforts into the main meal, not the dessert.

I also live in the hope that you're working on breaking the sweet habit and are making desserts an occasional thing, rather than a daily (or even twice-daily) inevitability. That being said, you might want a little something extra at the end of your meal from time to time. Here are a few ideas for fast low-carb end-of-the-meal treats:

Nuts and Sherry or Port

If you're not feeding children, simply passing a bowl of nuts in their shells, with nutcrackers (and plates for the shells), along with a little sherry or port, makes a nice end to a meal.

Cheese

Cheese for dessert may sound strange to sugar-addicted Americans, but it's an old European custom. I'd never tried this until I went on the Low-Carb High Life Cruise in 2001, and discovered that Carnival Cruise Lines has cheese on the dessert menu every night. My readers and I ended up ordering a cheese platter just about every night, and we all agreed that it made a nice—and very satisfying—end to a meal. If you have any empty corners after the meal, a little cheese is guaranteed to fill them right up. It's nicest to pass a slice or two of a few varieties—perhaps some sort of blue cheese, a soft cheese such as Camembert or Brie, and a firmer cheese such as Edam or Gouda. Add some Gruyère or Havarti, and perhaps a good strong cheddar, and you've got a winning assortment.

Coffee Drinks

If you're fond of coffee, try laying in a supply of either flavored coffees (the kind you actually brew, *not* the General Mills International Coffees, which contain sugar and other objectionable ingredients) and sugar-free coffee flavoring syrups (Da Vinci Sugar Free is probably the most widely available; look at your local gourmet coffee take-out joint, but Atkins and Monin O'Free are also fine). Combine these with some heavy cream, if you like, to make an endless array of coffee drinks. Use decaf if you find that caffeine after dinner keeps you awake.

Here are some ideas to jump-start your coffee creativity

⊕ Irish Coffee

I included this in *500 Low-Carb Recipes*, but it seemed too classic to omit here.

> 1 shot (1 1/2 ounces, 45 ml) Irish whiskey*
>
> 6 ounces hot coffee (170 ml)
>
> Splenda to taste
>
> Whipped cream (See Whipped Topping recipe, opposite page)

* You may as well use cheap, blended whiskey for this; use Jamieson's or Bushmill's and you'll make my husband cry.

The traditional glass for this is a stemmed Irish coffee mug, but I wouldn't bother running out and buying them, unless you're exceedingly fond of Irish coffee. Just put the shot of whiskey in a large mug, pour the coffee over it, add Splenda to taste, and top with a good dollop of whipped cream.

Yield: 1 serving. If you use 2 teaspoons of Splenda and a couple of tablespoons of whipped cream, you'll get just 2 grams of carbohydrates, no fiber, and no protein.

☺ Whipped Topping

This seems as good a place as any to repeat my favorite recipe for making whipped cream—the instant pudding in this recipe gives it a lovely, mild sweetness and a glorious texture. By the way, don't try to whip cream in your blender or food processor—it won't work. Use an electric mixer, an egg beater, or that old standby, the whisk. I think an electric mixer is best. Use this in coffee drinks, over berries, or anywhere else you think a little whipped cream might be nice. This recipe makes a lot; feel free to halve it.

> 1 cup heavy whipping cream, well chilled (250 ml)
>
> 1 tablespoon sugar-free vanilla instant pudding powder

Simply whip the two together until you have fluffy, gorgeous whipped cream. Don't overbeat, or you'll get sweet vanilla butter.

Yield: This is enough for a crowd—2 cups (500 ml), or 16 servings of 2 tablespoons, each with only a trace of carbohydrates, no fiber, and no protein.

Note: See the words "well chilled" after the cream in this recipe? That's because warm cream may well refuse to whip on you. Furthermore, your bowl and beaters shouldn't be warm, either. If they're fresh out of the dishwasher, chill them in the freezer for 5 to 10 minutes, or at the very least run cold water over them and then dry them before making your Whipped Topping.

⏲ Café Chantilly

This is a classic!

> 1 tablespoon cognac
>
> 4 ounces brewed coffee (120 ml)
>
> Unsweetened whipped cream (just whip chilled heavy cream by itself
> with an electric mixer)

Just stir the cognac into the coffee, top with a dollop of whipped cream, and serve.

Yield: 1 serving, with just 1 gram of carbohydrates, no fiber, and no protein.

❉ Each serving has only 65 calories!

⏲ Mexican Coffee

Traditionally this is made with pilloncillo sugar—Mexican brown sugar—
and milk, but that's too many carbs for us. Here's the reduced-carb version.

> 6 ounces brewed coffee (170 ml)
>
> 2 to 3 tablespoons heavy cream
>
> 2 teaspoons Splenda
>
> 2 drops blackstrap molasses*
>
> Tiny pinch ground cinnamon
>
> Tiny pinch ground cloves

* It helps to keep your blackstrap in a squeeze bottle. I buy my blackstrap in bulk
from my health food store and keep it in one of those "honey bears."

Pour the coffee, and stir in the cream, Splenda, and molasses. Sprinkle the spices
over the top and serve.

Yield: 1 serving, with 3 grams of carbohydrates, the merest trace of fiber,
and 1 gram of protein.

☻ Café Vienna

Coffee for chocolate lovers, or chocolate for coffee lovers.

> 6 ounces brewed coffee (170 ml)
>
> 2 tablespoons sugar-free chocolate coffee flavoring syrup
>
> 2 tablespoons heavy cream
>
> Tiny pinch ground cinnamon

Pour the coffee, stir in the chocolate syrup and heavy cream, dust the cinnamon over the top, and serve.

Yield: 1 serving. Assuming you use Atkins or Da Vinci coffee flavoring syrup (which are made with Splenda instead of polyols), this will have 2 grams of carbohydrates, a trace of fiber, and 1 gram of protein.

Note: If you'd like to spiff this up for company, used whipped cream (see Whipped Topping on page 231) instead of the plain heavy cream.

☻ Chocolate Orange Coffee

I came up with this one morning when my husband was out of cream for his coffee—it kept me from having to run out to the store before breakfast, and he loved it!

> 6 ounces brewed coffee (170 ml)
>
> 1 tablespoon sugar-free chocolate coffee flavoring syrup
>
> 1 or 2 drops orange extract

Pour the coffee and stir in the syrup and the extract. That's all!

Yield: 1 serving. Again assuming you use Atkins or Da Vinci brand syrup, you'll have just 1 gram of carbohydrates here, no fiber, and no protein.

Café Incontro

For adults only, of course!

> 6 ounces brewed coffee (170 ml)
>
> 1 scant shot dark rum (about 1 ounce, 30 ml)
>
> 2 teaspoons sugar-free chocolate coffee flavoring syrup
>
> Splenda to taste, if desired

Pour the coffee, add the rum, syrup, and Splenda, and serve. That's all!

Yield: 1 serving, with just 1 gram of carbohydrates (again, we're talking the Atkins or Da Vinci syrup), no fiber, and no protein. Add 0.5 grams of carbohydrates for each teaspoon of Splenda you add.

☻ Cinnamon Splenda Nuts

Okay, this isn't a coffee recipe, but it is a nice little nibble to pass around with coffee.

> 2 tablespoons butter
>
> 1 cup shelled walnuts, pecans, or a combination of the two (120 g)
>
> 1 1/2 to 2 tablespoons Splenda
>
> 1/2 teaspoon cinnamon

Melt the butter in a heavy skillet over medium heat, then add the nuts. Cook for 5 to 6 minutes, stirring from time to time. Turn off the heat and immediately sprinkle the Splenda and cinnamon over the top, and stir to distribute. (If you wait for the nuts to cool, the Splenda doesn't stick nearly so well.) I like these best warm, although they're still quite nice when cooled.

Yield: 4 or 5 servings (remember, this is just a nibble). Assuming 4 servings, each will have 5 grams of carbohydrates and 2 grams of fiber, for a total of 3 grams of usable carbs and 5 grams of protein.

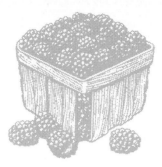

Fruit

Fruit desserts are an interesting question for the low-carb dieter. On the one hand, they're likely to have more carbohydrates than sugar-free commercially made stuff. On the other hand, they're likely to be far lower in calories—and calories still *do* count, at least some—and far, far more nutritious.

Which fruit you choose makes a big difference. A banana, for instance, will run you about 25 grams of carbohydrates, and a cup (150 g) of diced fresh pineapple has 19 grams. On the other hand, there are some fruits that are low enough in sugar to fit into our diets in moderation, and luckily for us, they're some of the most delectable. Here's a rundown of the lowest-sugar fruits, plus a few simple ideas for fruit desserts.

Apricots are a real bargain. One has just 3.9 grams of carbohydrates and 0.84 grams fiber, for a total of about 3 grams of usable carbs!

All of the berries are pretty low carb, and they make a terrific quick-and-easy dessert with either heavy cream or whipped cream. For that matter, you could eat them plain! By the way, berries are also among the most nutritious fruits available; you'll be getting a lot of benefit from the few carbs they add to your day.

- 1/2 cup (50g) **raspberries** has 7 grams of carbohydrates and 4.2 grams of fiber, for a total of just 2.8 grams of usable carbs.

- 1/2 cup (50g) **blackberries** has 9.2 grams of carbohydrates and 3.6 grams of fiber, for a total of 5.6 grams of usable carbs.

- 1/2 cup (50g) **strawberries** has 5.2 grams of carbohydrates and 2 grams of fiber, for a total of 3.2 grams of usable carbs.

- 1/2 cup (50g) **blueberries** has 10.2 grams of carbohydrates and 1.7 grams of fiber, for a total of 8.5 grams of usable carbs.

⊕ Strawberry Crunch Parfait

In their book *The GO-Diet*, Drs. Goldberg and O'Mara explain that plain yogurt has far fewer carbs than the label would indicate because most of the lactose in the milk has been converted to lactic acid by the yogurt bacteria. Accordingly, they say that we can count just 4 grams of carbohydrates per cup (225 ml) of plain yogurt. Reading this, I added yogurt back to my low-carb diet, and it's never caused weight gain or rebound hunger for me, so I think Goldberg and O'Mara are right! This recipe is so versatile—it makes a great dessert, a phenomenal quick breakfast, or a delicious and nutritious snack. Enjoy!

> 3 ripe strawberries
>
> 1 tablespoon plus 1/4 teaspoon Splenda
>
> 3/4 cup plain yogurt (170 ml)
>
> 1/2 teaspoon vanilla extract
>
> 2 tablespoons Cinnamon Splenda Nuts, chopped a bit (see page 234)
>> or 2 tablespoons Gram's Gourmet Flax 'n' Nut Crunchies (Vanilla Almond or Cinnamon Toast flavor) or other low-carb commercial granola-like product

Cut the green hulls off your strawberries, and slice them thinly into a dish. Sprinkle them with 1/4 teaspoon of the Splenda, and stir.

Combine the yogurt with the vanilla extract and the remaining tablespoon of Splenda, stirring well. Spoon over the strawberries. Top with the nuts or Flax 'n' Nut Crunchies, and devour!

Yield: 1 serving. Using the *GO-Diet's* carb count of 4 grams of carbohydrates per cup (225 ml) of plain yogurt, this has 12 grams of carbohydrates and 3 grams of fiber, for a total of 9 grams of usable carbs and 10 grams of protein.

Note: Feel free to substitute 1/4 cup (30 g) blueberries, blackberries, or raspberries, or even diced peaches. Make this in a clear glass dish, or even layer it in a parfait glass, and it'll look pretty enough for company.

☺ Fast Strawberry-Orange Sauce

This is especially nice for spiffing up a simple dessert for company, using up strawberries threatening to go bad in the refrigerator, or just because it's Tuesday.

> 1/2 cup strawberries—fresh, or frozen with no sugar added, thawed (50 g)
>
> 1 tablespoon Splenda
>
> 1/4 teaspoon orange extract

Assemble the ingredients in a food processor, and purée. Serve over sliced melon or sugar-free ice cream, or stir it into plain yogurt.

Yield: About 1/3 cup (75 ml), or 3 servings, each with 2 grams of carbohydrates and 1 gram of fiber, for a total of 1 gram of usable carbs and a trace of protein.

☺ Figs with Gorgonzola

It doesn't get any simpler or more elegant than this.

> 4 fresh, medium figs
> 1/4 cup crumbled Gorgonzola (30 g)
> 1/2 cup chopped walnuts (50 g)

Slice the figs in half, spread each half with a tablespoon of Gorgonzola, and sprinkle with 1/2 tablespoon chopped walnuts.

Yield: 4 servings of 2 halves, each with 12 grams of carbohydrates and 2 grams of fiber, for a total of 10 grams of usable carbs and 9 grams of protein.

Note: Some people like to broil the figs for a few minutes first.

I adore **pink grapefruit**, and since I've gone low-carb, it tastes really sweet to me! Grapefruit is higher in carbs than berries are, but still pretty okay: 1/2 medium grapefruit has 10.4 grams of carbohydrates and 1.4 grams of fiber, for a total of 9 grams of usable carbs. If you'd like to spiff up that grapefruit a little, you could sprinkle it with Splenda, or, as many people have suggested to me, Brown Sugar Twin. Personally, I drizzle my grapefruit with 1/4 teaspoon blackstrap molasses, which adds 1 scant gram of carbohydrates. I love the warm brown flavor of the molasses contrasted with the cool, sharp flavor of the grapefruit.

☺ Broiled Grapefruit

This is a classic sort of recipe.

> 1/2 grapefruit
> 1/2 teaspoon butter (optional)
> Splenda
> A touch of blackstrap molasses, if you like
> Ground cinnamon (optional)

Loosen the sections of the grapefruit by running a sharp, thin-bladed knife around each one. Sprinkle with the sweetener of your choice, plus cinnamon if you like, and broil a few inches (centimeters) from the flame for 10 minutes.

Yield: 1 serving, with 10.4 grams of carbohydrates and 1.4 grams of fiber, for a total of 9 grams of usable carbs from the grapefruit. Splenda has 0.5 grams of carbohydrates per teaspoon. Blackstrap has 1 gram of carbohydrates per 1/4 teaspoon—and it's so strong-flavored you won't want to use more than this!

Note: Some people like to cut the white core out and put butter in there.

Melon is a great low-carb dessert, and it's very nutritious. If you'd like to fancy it up a bit, sprinkle it with a little lime juice mixed with Splenda and ginger to taste, or top it with the Fast Strawberry Orange Sauce (see page 237)—but it's really a fine dessert as-is.

- 1/8 of a medium **cantaloupe** has 8.4 grams of carbohydrates and 0.8 grams of fiber, for a total of 7.6 grams of usable carbs.

- 1/8 of a medium **honeydew** has 9.2 grams of carbohydrates and 0.6 grams of fiber, for a total of 8.6 grams of usable carbs.

- 1 cup (250 g) of frozen **melon balls** has 8 grams of carbohydrates and 0.7 grams of fiber, for a total of 7.3 grams of usable carbs.

- 1 cup (250 g) diced **watermelon** has 11 grams of carbohydrates and 0.8 grams of fiber, for a total of 10.2 grams of usable carbs.

- One medium-size **nectarine** has 11.8 grams of carbohydrates and 1.6 grams of fiber, for a total of 10.2 grams of usable carbs.

- One medium **peach** has 11.1 grams of carbohydrates and 2 grams of fiber, for a total of 9.1 grams of usable carbs.

- One medium **plum** has 13.1 grams of carbohydrates and 1.5 grams of fiber, for a total of 11.6 grams of usable carbs.

- 1 medium fresh **fig** has 9.6 grams of carbohydrates and 1.6 grams of fiber, for a total of 8 grams of usable carbs.

☺ Speedy Low-Carb Peach Melba

This is a short-cut, no-sugar-added version of a very famous dessert—and it's scrumptious! You can use fresh peaches in this, if you'd prefer, but unlike the frozen ones, you'll have to peel and slice them, which may take you over the 15-minute time limit.

> 2 cups frozen, sliced, no-sugar-added peaches (500 g)
>
> 1/4 cup lemon juice (50 ml)
>
> 1/4 teaspoon orange extract
>
> 1/2 cup Splenda (50 g)
>
> 1 cup raspberries—fresh or frozen with no sugar added (120 g)
>
> 4 tablespoons toasted slivered almonds (optional)

Don't bother to thaw the frozen peaches. Put them in a microwaveable bowl, mix together 2 tablespoons of the lemon juice, the orange extract, and half of the Splenda, and pour it over them. Cover (I just lay a plate on top) and microwave on High for 5 to 7 minutes, or until tender right through.

While the peaches are poaching, put the raspberries, the remaining 2 tablespoons of lemon juice, and the remaining Splenda in your food processor with the S-blade in place. Pulse a few times until everything is puréed together.

When the peaches are done, divide between 4 small serving dishes, and divide the raspberry sauce between them. Sprinkle each dish with a tablespoon of almonds, if desired. Serve.

Yield: 4 servings, each with 17 grams of carbohydrates and 4 grams of fiber, for a total of 13 grams of usable carbs and 1 gram of protein. Add the optional almonds and each serving has 19 grams of carbohydrates and 5 grams of fiber, for a total of 14 grams of usable carbs and 3 grams of protein.

✻ This also has a mere 68 calories, every one of them nutritious.

Note: Now, this is not the traditional way to serve Peach Melba—the traditional way would include a scoop of vanilla ice cream. You could do this, of course, using one of the no-sugar-added ice creams, or Atkins Endulge (see page 241), but since this is already in the upper range of the low-carb recipe spectrum, I'd probably only do this for a very special occasion. You could also serve this with vanilla yogurt—see the Strawberry Crunch Parfait recipe (see page 236) for how-tos—and add only about 2.5 grams of carbs per 1/2 cup (120 ml) of yogurt.

> **Tip:** Feel free to make the raspberry sauce all by itself—it's great over melon, stirred into plain yogurt, or as an elegant quick dessert when combined with no-sugar ice cream.

Purchased Low-Carb Sweets

Low-carbohydrate chocolate or other sugar-free candy. This stuff gets better all the time and is now widely available. Since sugar-free candy is polyol-sweetened, it does technically have carbs in it, but the amount that most of you will absorb will be quite low. Still, both because of the possibility of more carb absorption than the labels let on and because of possible gastric distress, go easy, okay? My husband and I will often split a 1.5 ounce (40 g) sugar-free dark chocolate bar for dessert; this strikes me as plenty.

Sugar-free cocoa, made from mix. Read the labels on all the brands available at your grocery store—in mine, Swiss Miss Diet is the lowest in carbs, at 4 grams per cup (100 g).

No-Sugar-Added Ice Cream. The no-sugar ice cream is pretty darned good. My favorite is the brand called Dreyer's in the West and Edy's in the East, but Breyer's also makes one, and my grocery store even has a house brand of no-sugar-added ice cream. This stuff does still have usable, absorbable carbs in it—the lactose in the milk it was made from—so go *easy*. A "serving" is 1/2 cup (120 g), not a half a carton! The carb counts vary some, so *read your labels*.

Atkins Endulge Super Premium Ice Cream. I list this separately because it's somewhat different from the grocery store brands of no-sugar ice cream that I've tried. On the one hand, I don't think it tastes as good as Edy's or Breyer's, and it's more expensive. On the other hand, Endulge Ice Cream has two inestimable virtues: It's *far* lower in carbohydrates than the grocery store brands—about half the carbs of Edy's and Dreyer's—and it comes in single serving cups, a strong preventive to over indulgence. And it does taste good enough.

No-Sugar-Added Ice Pops. The Popsicle company makes a sugar-free variety, and they're among your lowest-carb prepared desserts—just 3 grams per pop and only 15 calories. So if you're a Popsicle fan, your dessert problems are solved! They're available in two assortments, either orange, cherry and grape, or the new tropical flavors, Caribbean fruit punch, Hawaiian pineapple, and tropical orange.

No-Sugar-Added Fudge Pops. No-sugar-added Fudgsicles taste just like the Fudgsicles of your youth—really, they do. Looking at the Popsicle company Website, they say these have 19 grams of carbohydrates and 1 gram of fiber per serving, which sounds like you're going to get a prohibitive 18 grams of carbs. But 3 grams are "sugar alcohols," aka polyols, so you can subtract them out, too, leaving 15 grams. Then you take a look at the "serving size"—which is two pops, not one. So if you eat one pop—which is what I'd be likely to do—you'll get 7.5 grams of usable carbs. And *that* fits into your low-carb diet!

There are also store brands of sugar-free fudge pops around; I know that Kroger—the biggest grocery chain in the United States—has one. Make sure to read the labels to find the true usable carb count, and don't forget to look at the serving size.

Sugar-Free Gelatin. It takes more than 15 minutes to make gelatin, if you count the chilling time, but Jell-O, for one, makes prepared sugar-free gelatin in plastic cups with peel-off tops; look for them under the name "Jell-O Snacks." If you like gelatin, this could be a handy item to keep in the pantry.

Sugar-Free Instant Pudding. Mix this with half heavy cream, half water to eliminate half of the carbs that using milk would add. If you do this before sitting down to dinner and set it in the refrigerator to chill, it should be at least passably thickened by the time dessert rolls around. According to my calculations, using the sugar-free instant pudding I have in the pantry, this would come to 8 grams of carbohydrates per serving.

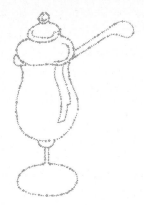

Sodas or Floats

These are American classics, and are really quick and simple to make. You may, of course, use any flavor of no-sugar-added ice cream and any flavor of diet soda to make floats. These are just a few popular combinations. You can also use one of the sugar-free coffee-flavoring syrups plus seltzer or club soda in place of the diet soda, if you'd like to get really creative.

⊕ Root Beer Float

My sister keeps IBC Sugar-Free Root Beer and Dreyer's Vanilla No-Sugar-Added Ice Cream in the house for this purpose and this purpose alone.

> 1 small scoop vanilla no-sugar-added ice cream or 1 serving Atkins Endulge
> Super Premium Ice Cream, vanilla flavor
> 1 can or bottle sugar-free root beer, well chilled

Put the ice cream in a large glass or mug, and pour the root beer over it. Serve with straws and a long-handled spoon.

Yield: 1 serving; the carb count will depend on your brand of no-sugar-added ice cream.

�---☉ Chocolate Float

If you can get chocolate-flavored diet soda in your region, this is a nice variant of the Root Beer Float.

> 1 small scoop vanilla no-sugar-added ice cream or 1 serving Atkins Endulge
> Super Premium Ice Cream, vanilla flavor
> 1 can sugar-free chocolate-fudge flavored soda, well chilled

Put the ice cream in a large glass or mug, and pour the soda over it. Serve with a straw and a long-handled spoon.

Yield: 1 serving; the carb count will depend on your brand of no-sugar-added ice cream.

Note: Canfield's makes diet chocolate-fudge flavored soda. If you can't find it in a local grocery store, there are several Websites that sell it. Be aware, however, that this is one of those love-it-or-hate-it products. Faygo also makes a chocolate soda.

☉ Dreamsicle Float

If you were a fan of Dreamsicles as a kid, you'll love this float!

> 1 small scoop no-sugar-added vanilla ice cream or 1 serving Atkins Endulge
> Super Premium Ice Cream, vanilla flavor
> 1 can sugar-free orange soda, well chilled

Put the ice cream in a large glass or mug, and pour the soda over it. Serve with a straw and a long-handled spoon.

Yield: 1 serving; the carb count will depend on your brand of no-sugar-added ice cream.

☺ Farmer's Soda

Simpler than a float and a bit lower carb.

> 1/4 cup heavy cream (50 ml)
>
> 1 can sugar-free soda, flavor of your choice, well chilled

Simply pour the cream into the bottom of a large glass, and pour the soda over it.

Yield: 1 serving, with 3 grams of carbohydrates, no fiber, and no protein.

Index

ALSO BY DANA CARPENDER

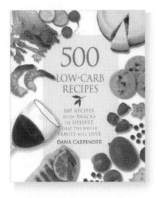

500 Low~Carb Recipes
by Dana Carpender

ISBN 1-931412-06-5
$19.95 (£9.99)
Paperback, 500 pages
Available wherever books are sold

Okay, you've finally done it. You've gone low-carb! And no matter which one of the many low-carbohydrate diets you've chosen, you've discovered the joys of weight loss without hunger, not to mention energy that never seems to quit, and rapidly improving health.

Just one little problem: If you have to face one more day of eggs for breakfast, tuna salad for lunch, and a burger without the bun for dinner, you're going to scream. Worse, you're going to order a pizza!

Rejoice, my low-carb friend. Help is here; you hold it in your hands. In this book you'll find options galore. You'll find dozens upon dozens of new things to do with your protein foods and vegetables and you'll find recipes for foods you thought you'd never, ever be able to eat on your low-carb diet:

- Cinnamon Raisin Bread • Feta-Spinach Salmon Roast
- Sour Cream Coffee Cake • Obscenely Rich Shrimp
- Chocolate Mousse to DIE For • Mom's Chocolate Chip Cookies
- Mockahlua Cheesecake • French Toast • Heroin Wings
- Sugar-Free Ketchup and Barbecue Sauce

You'll also learn more about how to count carbs and read labels, as well as get an overview of low-carb ingredients. You'll get the lowdown on all those new low-carb specialty products flooding the market. And, of course, you get 14 chapters of recipes, covering everything from Hors d'Oeuvres, Snacks, and Party Nibbles, to Breads, Muffins, Cereals and Other Grainy Things.

You'll find cookies, cakes, and other sweets. Plus more recipes for main dishes and side dishes than you'll ever be able to eat your way through—everything from down-home cooking to ethnic fare; from quick-and-easy weeknight meals to knock-their-socks-off party food. So say goodbye to boredom, and hello to exciting low-carb meals every day! Whether you're a kitchen novice or a gourmet chef, you'll find dozens of recipes to suit your tastes, budget, and lifestyle.

ALSO BY DANA CARPENDER

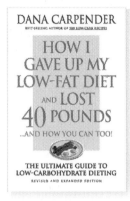

How I Gave Up My Low-Fat Diet and Lost 40 Pounds

by Dana Carpender

ISBN 1-59233-040-1
$14.95 (£9.99)
Paperback, 312 pages
Available wherever books are sold

It's time to go low carb! Low-carbohydrate diets burn off twice the fat of low-fat or low-calorie diets, and they do it without making you starve. Here's the lowdown on how and why low-carbohydrate dieting works, not just for weight loss, but for dramatic health improvement. Without using boring, confusing medical jargon, I'll show you surprising research proving that carbohydrates, not fat, are the biggest culprit in causing diseases like diabetes, cancer, and coronary artery disease. Then I'll explain to you not one, but more than a half-a-dozen different approaches to cutting the carbs, and give you the information you need to mix-and-match these plans to come up with a low-carbohydrate diet you can live with for the rest of your long and healthy life.

So c'mon! Let me show you how to:

- Lose weight without hunger!
- Have the energy of a kid again!
- Eat more wonderful, real food than you ever thought possible!

All the while improving your cholesterol and triglycerides, lowering your blood pressure, and cutting your risk of diabetes and cancer. Let me tell you *How I Gave Up My Low-Fat Diet and Lost 40 Pounds . . . and How You Can Too!*